PRAISE FOR *REVOLUTION OF THE SOUL*

"Seane Corn took me by the hand and led me into so much more than a yoga practice. She guided me through my body, into my mind, and into an appreciation for the sound of breathing, the people around me, and for my own two feet. She is a gift."
SALLY FIELD
Academy Award®-winning actor and *New York Times* bestselling author of *In Pieces*

"Holy hell, do we need a worldwide love revolution! After reading *Revolution of the Soul*, I am more convinced than ever that we can have it: but only if we begin with ourselves. *Revolution of the Soul* is heart-wrenchingly vulnerable, relentlessly honest, and refreshingly hilarious. With every personal story, Seane wrangles the power of yoga down from the clouds and into our ordinary relationships, hardships, and bodies. Then she shows us how to use that power to heal ourselves and the world. Seane is a master teacher, one of my favorite human beings, and a hell of a writer. I am a better person for having read this book."
GLENNON DOYLE
founder of Together Rising and author of the #1 *New York Times* bestseller *Love Warrior*

"Seane's passionate, tough, compelling, honorable, healing dharma story will touch your heart . . . and inspire the real yogi in you."
JACK KORNFIELD, PHD
author of *A Path with Heart*

"Seane Corn is a wise and beautiful woman, articulating elegantly modern teachings that emerge from ancient truths. Her book is a gift to all of us."
MARIANNE WILLIAMSON
acclaimed lecturer, activist, and *New York Times* bestselling author of *A Return to Love, Healing the Soul of America, Tears to Triumph,* and *A Politics of Love*

"This book is everything that Seane is as a teacher and person in life: authentic, raw, honest, irreverent, self-aware, and joyously inspirational. *Revolution of the Soul* is filled with humor, hope, and the direct transmissions of love, grace, and magic that you come to expect from Seane when you enter her class. If you know her work, on and off the mat, you will hear her powerful voice on every page and feel comforted by her guidance. For those of you who are being introduced to Seane's work for the first time, you are in for a heart-opening, ass-kicking, and soul-stirring ride. Enjoy every moment. For it will blow your heart wide open and invite you into a movement of inner and outer change that can heal this world toward peace."
NAOMI WATTS
Academy Award®-nominated actor, film producer

"Reading *Revolution of the Soul* is like having the most amazing conversation with your wisest, funniest, and kindest friend. Seane's honesty and vulnerability will inspire you to get real and heal! She shares beautiful teachings and practices that will help you free yourself from limiting beliefs and effect change from a place of love."
GABBY BERNSTEIN
#1 *New York Times* bestselling author of *The Universe Has Your Back*

"A wondrous kaleidoscope of stories told with grit, humor, and humility, *Revolution of the Soul* will inspire you to take your practice off the mat and into the world—and show you how."
VALARIE KAUR, JD
founder of The Revolutionary Love Project

"It is hard for me to imagine anyone else could write this book other than Seane Corn. It is laced with deep wisdom that was born out of the challenges and tribulations of Seane's life. In other words, it is real! And the realness of her path means this wisdom can be learned and applied by all of us as we walk this crazy path of being alive in today's world. I am grateful for this modern woman's modern wisdom."

CONGRESSMAN TIM RYAN
Ohio, author of *Healing America*

"Seane was my first yoga teacher 25 years ago. Back then she was a passionate and magnetic teacher just finding her voice. Seane proves what time and practice can do. In *Revolution of the Soul*, Seane uses that voice—and opens her own soul—to reveal herself to be a wise and profound woman, sharing all she has learned on her journey as a yogi, woman, and citizen of the Earth. This book is accessible, poetic, and full of love and hope, and it provides the necessary tools for the reader to do their own soul's work and explore what it means to be in service to the world today."

DEBRA MESSING
actress, activist, and mother

"In this insightful and integrated book, Seane Corn journeys into the depth of essential wisdom that can be found on the yoga mat. Drawing connections from classic ancient teachings and physical practices to modern-day realities, she presents a roadmap from abstract theory to in-your-life application. She boldly confronts issues of privilege, race, and justice that yogis and meditators too often bypass, starting where it matters: from the inside out. Seane goes beyond the lip service that our liberation is bound together and offers up her own journey—backsteps and all—as an invitation for each and every one of us to walk our own path of liberation, too."

REV. ANGEL KYODO WILLIAMS
Sensei, author of *Radical Dharma*, and founder of Transformative Change

"Thank you, Seane, for courageously digging deep to bring forth with compassion, humor, and wisdom the stories and healing tools of your own personal journey to transform the most difficult shadow issues and traumas into a revolution of the soul on behalf of all. Thank you for inspiring and empowering the world with the way you lead with love and embody activism from the heart."

SHIVA REA
founder of the Samudra Global School for Living Yoga and author of *Tending the Heart Fire*

"One of the traditions that I study asks, 'If it's not practical, how can it be spiritual?' In *Revolution of the Soul*, Seane takes the ancient wisdom and practices from yogic traditions and transforms them into a practical way to inquire into our everyday lives. It invites us into the introspection of how to see more clearly and love more deeply through relevant, honest, and beautifully polished reflections that inform and reveal things we don't even know that we don't know. I LOVE this book! Quite frankly, I personally deem *Revolution of the Soul* necessary and required reading for all on the path of yoga . . . especially for yogis in the Western world."

R. NIKKI MYERS
founder of Y12SR: The Yoga of 12-Step Recovery

"Love this book. Like Seane herself, the message is direct, honest, funny, heartfelt, and filled with wisdom that can help all of us, except me, do better, be better, and work toward creating a healthier and more peaceful planet for all."

LARRY DAVID
actor, writer, director, producer of *Curb Your Enthusiasm* and *Seinfeld*

"Only Seane Corn could write a sweeping, insightful, spiritual manifesto that still feels so relatable and grounded—so . . . gritty. *Revolution of the Soul* is for anyone who wants to feel a little more connected to the world around them, to the people in their lives, and to themselves."

KATE FAGAN
sports journalist, author of *What Made Maddy Run* and *The Reappearing Act*, and cohost of *Free Cookies*

"Seane Corn's account of her discovery of yoga is positively riveting, and it is paired with a systematic description of the path—as it gradually unfolds itself in her life. Corn writes like a skilled novelist—building suspense and quietly drawing the grateful reader into an irresistible world. I simply could not put this book down. It is raw, honest, moving, hilarious, and oh-so-human. I predict that many, many people will find themselves in the pages of this story, and will find here too the very soul of yoga."

STEPHEN COPE
scholar-in-residence, Kripalu Center for Yoga & Health, and author of many bestselling books on yoga and meditation, including *Yoga and the Quest for the True Self* and *The Great Work of Your Life*

"My friend and sister has written a hilarious, holy, raw, deep, and essential book about life, not just yoga. Her voice, which I have been blessed to know for 20 years, is rich, astonishingly honest, messy, and messianic with promise and hope of transformative healing for all beings. It is replete with practical guidance for rolling out our yoga mats, literally and metaphorically, and stepping onto our paths of radical self-inquiry, discovery, and accountability, all for the ultimate purpose of being in healthy, honorable, and sustainable service to our fellows and our world. Read this book!"

ASHLEY JUDD
actor, activist, and *New York Times* bestselling author of *All That Is Bitter and Sweet*

"Seane has written a powerful book about the connection between the inner work of personal growth and the outer work of social justice. It speaks to the ways we create, and can heal, from the attitudes and ideas that separate us from each other, this planet, and our highest nature. I appreciate the timeliness of this message and the honest and straightforward way in which Seane delivers it."

DAVID GEFFEN
philanthropist, producer, and cofounder of Asylum Records, Geffen Records, and DreamWorks SKG

"I have known Seane as a teacher and, more importantly, as a dear friend for over 25 years. This book is fully the woman I know, trust, and love. Every word, every story, is filled with truth bombs and gorgeous wisdom. But what makes this book compelling is that Seane is a natural-born storyteller, and her life lessons read like a page-burner fiction. Except they are all true. These stories, like Seane herself, are raw, funny, deeply transparent, and unafraid to confront the power of our shared humanity and spirit. Seane shares them in service to help us relate to the challenges of our own life experience. Beyond the narratives she shares, what makes *Revolution of the Soul* so unique are the spiritual and psychological tools that accompany each story, helping us to unpack the deeper transformational wisdom that can lead to both personal and collective healing and peace. I couldn't recommend this special book more. It is a game changer and should be read by all."

ELIZABETH BERKLEY LAUREN
actress, teen girl advocate, and *New York Times* bestselling author of *Ask Elizabeth*

"Seane does what so many authors have tried and failed: she writes like she speaks. Her book is an intimate conversation at the kitchen table—raw, hilarious, profound, and human. Her story reflects back to us the many parts of ourselves that are learning and growing and reminds us that a revolution of the soul is possible for each and every one of us. This book is provocative and inspiring—just like Seane. Get it."

KERRI KELLY
founder of CTZNWELL
and host of *CTZN Podcast*

"Seane saved many lives, including mine. Read this book, and she'll help you too."

BOBBY SHRIVER
activist and cofounder of ONE, (RED), and the *Very Special Christmas* record project

"A brilliant piece of work that is grounded in honesty and vulnerability. Seane Corn takes bold moves by sharing her experiences and lessons on activism and service through the lens of yoga. This text is essential for yoga teachers, practitioners, and anyone interested in the connections between liberation, service, and yoga. Seane's book is right on time and is a must-read for anyone excited to harness and understand the power within in order to mindfully impact social change."

CHELSEA JACKSON ROBERTS, PHD, E-RYT
cofounder of Red Clay Yoga

"*Revolution of the Soul* is raw, uncensored, and in your face. It gives you the invitation and opportunity to unpack your traumas with the support of yoga. Seane lights the way with her own personal journey on this path of growth and evolution."

EDDIE MODESTINI
founder of Maya Yoga

"The world knows Seane Corn as a healer, a teacher, and a leader of the revolution to awaken others to their higher potential. In this book, they will get to know her as a person—a person who faces all the same doubts and fears that we all do. In *Revolution of the Soul*, she courageously allows us to witness her darkest moments and inspiring triumphs, while also sharing the tools of transformation she's cultivated from over 30 years of dedicated practice—tools that can heal, awaken, reconnect, and move all of us toward transcendence and peace." **DAMIEN ECHOLS**
New York Times bestselling
author of *Life After Death*,
Yours for Eternity,
and *High Magick*

"In *Revolution of the Soul*, Seane courageously reveals her own emotional journeys—exploring the many facets of truth, unfolding them from the darkness and pain. Seane goes after rinsing the gritchy places in the soul and gives the reader her real-life examples of how to use yoga principles to move victoriously through the facades, entrapments, terrors, shadows, and successes of life. I love that. I respect Seane for her relentless dismantling of her own facades, thus earning living from her authentic self. That accomplishment is rare and wondrous. Seane Corn is a great guide to becoming your own best advocate, as well as learning to care enough to be an activist healing our ailing world. Thank you, Seane, for putting your experiences and teaching into this book. You have just added another great gift to our people." **ANA TIGER FORREST**
creatrix of Forrest Yoga, medicine woman,
and author of *Fierce Medicine*

"With authenticity as real and raw as giving birth, this book will tear your heart out and hand it back to you busted wide open. Truth shines like a beacon from every page, while the sacred and profane are elevated to a whole new level beyond separation. Take this exquisitely personal journey through Heaven and Hell to embrace the true heart of yoga as pure, passionate, and potent LOVE. Seane has written a book I will carry in my heart and out to the world."

ANODEA JUDITH, PHD
author of *Eastern Body, Western Mind*,
The Global Heart Awakens, and *Wheels of Life*

"This radical and real gem of a book is a spiritual pilgrimage through the desert of life's difficulties to the holiness of your own beautiful heart and soul. Thank you, Seane Corn, for showing us what it takes sometimes to become a true, deep, and seasoned human being."

KATHERINE WOODWARD THOMAS
New York Times bestselling author of *Calling
in "The One"* and *Conscious Uncoupling*

"This is the book I have been longing to offer psychotherapy clients and yoga students alike as required reading. Seane not only reveals how to apply both what is practical and mystical about the path of yoga, but also masterfully describes how her practice transformed her thought systems, maladaptive behaviors, and emotional wounds. Seane invites us into her inner world through hard-won humility and a decades-long welcoming and absolving of her own symptoms. Anyone who has suffered from anxiety; has been the survivor of physical, emotional, or sexual abuse, mood, substance, or eating disorders; or is struggling from any other symptoms rooted in trauma will be offered hope and shepherded into transformation through this book. *Revolution of the Soul* is worth thousands of dollars of time on the therapist's couch. Through a powerful framework of lived experience and ancient teachings, Seane illuminates yoga's medicine to ameliorate suffering and create well-being in mind, body, and a revolutionized soul. No matter where we are in our own awakening, this book is a gift to us all." **MELODY MOORE, PHD, RYT**
psychologist and founder of
the Embody Love Movement

"For anyone seeking greater mindfulness or something more divine, Seane Corn is an inspiring companion. In this book, she interweaves a captivating memoir of self-awakening that starts in the sex-drugs-and-rock-and-roll days of New York City in the 1980s with the spiritual and practical lessons she learned on her path toward becoming a renowned yoga instructor, a passionate advocate of healing, and a dedicated international activist. Her journey—and its evocative telling—offers valuable guidance and encouragement for those on their own quest." **DAVID CORN**
Washington bureau chief of
Mother Jones and *New York Times* bestselling
author of *Russian Roulette* and *Showdown*

"*Revolution of the Soul* is not your mother's yoga book, and Seane Corn is not your average spiritual teacher. If you are looking for rainbows and unicorns, look somewhere else. But if you are looking for the real deal—the beautiful yet hard truth of inner change and transformation—then read on. Because this book delivers. It challenges the meager stories we cart around in our heads and asks us to replace them with bigger and bolder versions of ourselves and our lives together as friends and citizens. Thank you, Seane Corn, for being so brave and wise."
ELIZABETH LESSER
cofounder of Omega Institute and author of
Broken Open, Marrow, and *The Seeker's Guide*

"The courage in this book is in Seane's vulnerability, in not having all the answers. Seane doesn't show us all the places she's done amazing work; she shows how she learned that she had work to do. In white Western yoga circles, I too often see yoga being used to avoid discomfort. I witness teachers glossing over violence and suffering, I hear people saying that yoga shouldn't be political. As someone who has journeyed alongside Seane, I know the depth of her practice and the depth of her seeking. I encourage you to travel with her through this book, as I have, and learn from the teacher my marginalized, traumatized body trusts with everything in me." **TEO DRAKE**
cofounder of the Transforming Hearts Collective

"In this groundbreaking book, Seane takes us through a deeply personal journey of trauma and transformation. Her stories will move you to tears; they will break your heart open and offer you a gem that you can take into your own life. Seane's raw vulnerability and profound grace is important medicine in these days where so many of us are overwhelmed and isolated. Seane reveals her humanity in a way that will transport you into a world of healing and possibility."
HALA KHOURI, MA, SEP, E-RYT
cofounder of Off the Mat, Into the World®

SEANE CORN

REVOLUTION
OF THE SOUL

AWAKEN TO LOVE THROUGH RAW TRUTH, RADICAL HEALING, AND CONSCIOUS ACTION

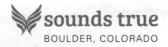 sounds true
BOULDER, COLORADO

Sounds True
Boulder, CO 80306

Published 2019

Book design by Beth Skelley

Seane Corn triangle logo © 2019 Gayheart Design

All lines from "Footnote to Howl" from *Collected Poems 1947–1980* by Allen Ginsberg.
Copyright © 1955 by Allen Ginsberg. Reprinted by permission of HarperCollins Publishers.

"Footnote to Howl" by Allen Ginsberg, currently in *Collected Poems 1947–1997*.
Copyright © 2006 Allen Ginsberg LLC. Used by permission of The Wylie Agency LLC.

"A Very Cellular Song" words and music by Mike Heron. Copyright © 1968 (renewed)
Warner-Tamerlane Publishing Corp. All rights reserved. Used by permission of Alfred Music.

Printed in Canada
Printed on FSC-compliant paper

Library of Congress Cataloging-in-Publication Data

Names: Corn, Seane, author.
Title: Revolution of the soul : awaken to love through raw truth, radical healing, and conscious action /
    Seane Corn.
Description: Boulder, CO : Sounds True, Inc., 2019.
Identifiers: LCCN 2018055546 (print) | LCCN 2019018267 (ebook) | ISBN 9781622039180 (ebook) |
    ISBN 9781622039173 (hardback)
Subjects: LCSH: Corn, Seane. | Yoginis—United States—Biography. | Yoga.
Classification: LCC B132.Y6 (ebook) | LCC B132.Y6 C646 2019 (print) | DDC 181/.45—dc23
LC record available at https://lccn.loc.gov/2018055546

10 9 8 7 6 5 4 3 2 1

To my sainted mother, Alice, my most beloved angel.
Thank you Ma for guiding my soul the way you have.
You encouraged me to trust my path, and I soared
because I always knew you would catch my fall,
celebrate the lessons learned, help me laugh at the
weirdness of it all, and love me fiercely no matter what.
I honor you for the vibrant, steady, funny, badass, wild,
and wonderful woman you are and for the deep amazing
soul connection we share. I love you. This book is for you.

CONTENTS

Holy! Holy! Holy! Holy! Holy! Holy! Holy! Holy! Holy! Holy! Holy! Holy! Holy!
    Holy! Holy!
The world is holy! The soul is holy! The skin is holy! The nose is holy! The tongue and
    cock and hand and asshole holy!
Everything is holy! everybody's holy! everywhere is holy! everyday is in eternity!
    Everyman's an angel!
The bum's as holy as the seraphim! the madman is holy as you my soul are holy!
The typewriter is holy the poem is holy the voice is holy the hearers are holy the ecstasy
    is holy!
Holy Peter holy Allen holy Solomon holy Lucien holy Kerouac holy Huncke holy
    Burroughs holy Cassady holy the unknown buggered and suffering beggars holy the
    hideous human angels!
Holy my mother in the insane asylum! Holy the cocks of the grandfathers of Kansas!
Holy the groaning saxophone! Holy the bop apocalypse! Holy the jazzbands marijuana
    hipsters peace peyote pipes & drums!
Holy the solitudes of skyscrapers and pavements! Holy the cafeterias filled with the
    millions! Holy the mysterious rivers of tears under the streets!
Holy the lone juggernaut! Holy the vast lamb of the middleclass! Holy the crazy
    shepherds of rebellion! Who digs Los Angeles IS Los Angeles!
Holy New York Holy San Francisco Holy Peoria & Seattle Holy Paris Holy Tangiers
    Holy Moscow Holy Istanbul!
Holy time in eternity holy eternity in time holy the clocks in space holy the fourth
    dimension holy the fifth International holy the Angel in Moloch!
Holy the sea holy the desert holy the railroad holy the locomotive holy the visions holy
    the hallucinations holy the miracles holy the eyeball holy the abyss!
Holy forgiveness! mercy! charity! faith! Holy! Ours! bodies! suffering! magnanimity!
Holy the supernatural extra brilliant intelligent kindness of the soul!

ALLEN GINSBERG
"Footnote to Howl"

INTRODUCTION

HOLY IS RIGHT! What an intense and wild time to be alive. There is much conflict and division in our world, but as difficult as these times are, they are also exciting, invigorating, and abundant with possibility. People are speaking out and rising up. It's inspiring, it's hopeful and—when so many lives are at stake—utterly necessary. As musician and poet Patti Smith says, "The people have the power" to unite, organize, and create real social change. Change that benefits everyone. Change that leads to liberation, to Oneness, to God. And that power is love. That is the revolution of the soul. But how can we harness that power? How do we awaken to love? How do we honor, as Allen Ginsberg said, all moments, beings, and experiences as holy? It begins with our own spiritual evolution. It begins by embracing the holiness in our own ever-evolving consciousness.

I wrote *Revolution of the Soul* in part to inspire, and provide the tools for, anyone who desires to participate in creating a better world. My hope is that these pages will encourage you to look beyond your limited perceptions, and the stories the ego so carefully curates, so you can get to the truth of your soul. This book is intensely personal and, hopefully, universally applicable. Each chapter has a story from my own healing journey and spiritual path, accompanied by a vast array of teachings—both practical and spiritual—that I've been exposed to over the years, including traditional yoga philosophy, modern psychology, metaphysics, and social justice methodology. I use these teachings to unpack the deeper complexities of each story and how it can be applied to your own experience. As James Baldwin says, "In order to have a conversation with someone you have to reveal yourself."

This book demanded vulnerability and raw honesty in a way I hadn't expected and frankly, I wasn't so sure I wanted to comply, at least not publicly. But I quickly realized that I couldn't ask you to do the brave, messy inner work of transformative change and opt out myself. I couldn't ask for a revolution, then not show up! Therefore, as you will soon see, I chose to pull the veils back and expose the tender, hidden parts of my journey. I tried to model what it means to "do the work" of inside-out change without apology, without thinking that it should have been different than it was. The experience of unpacking certain aspects of my journey was humbling, to say the least, but also incredibly liberating. I hope the process can be that for you as well. I believe strongly that to heal the planet, we must be willing to heal the parts of ourselves that contribute to its suffering. Personal accountability is hard, but necessary. It's easy to tell the world to change its ways and values; it's another thing to have to change our own.

Therefore, to do the work, we must unwrap all of our stories—the highlights and the lowlights and the what-the-fucks—and take a long, loving look at each one of them. Why? So we can unearth the angels buried within the narratives and the teachers we've long forgotten—or refused to acknowledge—and repair any separation we've inadvertently caused within ourselves and toward others. Separation that may be blocking us from our deepest Self. To participate in the change we want to see in the world, we must investigate, learn from, and release everything that gets in our way. In other words, we must set a place at our heart's table for all that we are—our joys, sorrows, unprocessed emotions, and individual and ancestral traumas—so we can see, acknowledge, and love others for who they are. So that we can embrace the holiness within all. So that we may serve.

I hope that by sharing my stories with you, you'll be inspired to look at your own, unfiltered. You'll notice that I don't sugarcoat anything. My stories are raw, revealing, intimate, and very human at times. Yours may be, too; they'll definitely be unique. But I can almost guarantee if you commit to diving deeply into those narratives—and no editing allowed!—you'll uncover the key to breaking shame and discovering the origins of your own limiting beliefs and biases, and better understand myriad pathways that lead to unification . . . and to love.

That is our deepest work. We must commit to love—ourselves, each other, the planet, the light, and the shadow—each moment and every experience, and know, that in love, we are unified; we are whole. This is what leads to peace.

Part I of this book is about looking within, cultivating various traditional and contemporary tools for personal transformation—especially yoga—and taking responsibility for our own healing, awareness, and growth. This pathway, and the soulful exploration that guides it, leads to our spiritual maturation. The evolution of our soul. Personal development is essential, but it's only one part of the journey toward wholeness. Action must follow.

Part II expands our awareness beyond individual growth. It asks us to explore how, through radical accountability and compassionate, informed action, we can use what we've learned about ourselves to change this world and to understand the interdependency that demands we do so. It means being a co-conspirator on the path committed to the freedom and rights of all beings and developing the skills to approach social change and justice through the framework of self-responsibility, understanding, and love for one reason only: because our collective liberation depends on it.

Clearly, we have work to do, work that will heal and change the world from the inside out. That's what this book is about. Our evolution *is* the revolution, a revolution that will hopefully lead to the awakened leadership we need—and we need it now more than ever.

Thank you for letting me share a bit of my own journey and soul's work with you. I hope it inspires you to continue your own inner work and motivates you to join the revolution of compassionate and activated souls who will love this world into peace.

So, let's begin our revolution by setting an intention and connecting with that which binds us all in love.

Dear Spirit,

May the reading of this book be an opportunity for healing, awakening, and remembering to occur in body, mind, and spirit. May we see beyond our own stories, letting go of everything we think we know and embracing spiritual perception, which is limitless and beyond reason, seeing all moments and all souls as holy. May we have the strength to do our inner work so we may confront our limiting beliefs, mature our awareness, and expand our intuitive knowing. May we be fearless in our pursuit for personal awakening and open ourselves to the God within and the God within all. May we love bigger, bolder, and more brilliantly than we ever thought possible; heal the divisions that exist; and have the courage to expose that which no longer serves our light. And as we heal, as we awaken, and as we work to evolve our soul, may we understand what it is that binds and bonds us all as One, in God and in love. May we step into the Mystery, and into this revolution, with our hearts open, our minds clear, and our souls emblazoned in Grace. May God lead, love inspire, and our actions fuel each other, this nation, and our world into peace.

Amen. Shalom. Salaam. Namaste. Aho. Shanti. Peace. Om.

PART I

EVOLUTION OF THE SOUL

The personal revolution is far more difficult,
and is the first step in any revolution.

MICHAEL FRANTI
musician, filmmaker, activist

FINDING GOD IN HEAVEN

MY FIRST LESSONS in spirituality and yoga had nothing to do with a mat, but everything to do with waking up. They included angels, seeing God, and being in Heaven. But, believe me, not the way you may think.

A few weeks after graduating high school in my hometown of Pompton Lakes, New Jersey, I packed up and made my way to New York City's East Village, the place I would call home for the next eight years. The East Village in the '80s was dirty, dangerous, and phenomenally exciting for a curious mind and a free spirit like mine. It was eclectic and alive with young punks, old Eastern European immigrants, innovative artists, gang members, squatters, and homeless people living in tents in Tompkins Square Park. I lived on Avenue B, between 12th and 13th Streets. Drugs, like heroin and crack, were sold in the bodega below me, but believe it or not, I always felt safe. It was common knowledge to live where the drugs were sold because that's not where they were used. Buyers had to go a block or two away to use so they wouldn't draw attention to the dealer. Dealers didn't want any trouble with the residents either, so they'd make an effort to learn our names and keep an eye out on the neighborhood.

In the eight years I lived in New York City, I worked as a coat check, hostess, waitress, bartender, and doorperson in well-known nightclubs, including MK, Grolier

Club, Tunnel, Cat Club, Limelight, Paradise, and Peggy Sue's, and in gay clubs like Shescape, Heaven, and the Clit Club. I earned a great living and made wonderful friends, many of whom I still have today. Odds are if you were partying in NYC in the mid '80s to early '90s, I probably helped you get drunk, stoned, or laid!

Let's start in Heaven where I met Billy, the man who would become my dearest angel.

Heaven was an all-male gay sex club located in the rectory of an old church that served as a famous nightclub known as Limelight, where I worked tending bar. On any given night, I'd pull up on my motorcycle, a 1970 650cc Triumph, wearing a silver vinyl miniskirt; a vintage red, white, and blue leather jacket; and go-go boots, with my hair dyed blue-black, piled high in a bouffant tucked tightly under my helmet. I'd saunter into the club, punch in, and head to the disco, where I was stationed most evenings.

The disco was the heart of the club, and all night long, I could feel the pulse of the bass in my body as I served drinks for tips to young people with fluorescent mohawks or Madonna scarves tied up in their hair, their arms festooned with tattoos and adorned with rubber bracelets. Mostly I'd get an extra dollar or two per drink, but sometimes I'd score, and someone would slide me a small folded triangle of waxed paper filled with a line of cocaine. I would do a bump by sprinkling some on the back of my hand and snorting it without missing a beat. High above me in cages, drag queens and transgender women danced and teased the crowd below. Most nights I worked until 4 a.m., the sound pounding in my ears long after I left. I'd head out to Angelica's or the Warsaw diner for breakfast with my friends before sliding into bed at 7 a.m., hoping to get a little sleep as the coke still coursed through my system.

One night the beer tap got jammed, so I left my station at the bar and went looking for my manager, who I was told had been last seen heading out the doors toward the back of the club. Just through those doors was a steep climb of steps and on the wall an old brass plate that said "rectory," a visible reminder that this was once an active church. I grinned to myself as I started up the stairs. We're all going to hell.

I could hear dance music getting louder the closer I got to the top landing where red velvet ropes, attached to two brass stanchions, blocked my entrance. It was obvious there was a party going on, so I unhooked the rope and peeked inside. The party was wild, boisterous, and loud. I could see a large crowd of people dancing and was surprised. How could I have not known about this? Excited, I started through the doorway, but before I got my foot over the threshold, an arm reached out and blocked me. A large male bouncer I didn't recognize was staring back at me. He was wearing black leather pants, a leather vest, and a police-like cap and nothing else. His very hairy chest glistened with sweat. His nipples were pierced and connected together with a silver chain. Another thicker chain that hung straight down his chest disappeared into his leather pants.

"Oh, hey," I said, startled by his sudden presence, "I work here. I'm Seane. I'm looking for Rick."

"Don't care. You can't come in. No women allowed."

"What are you talking about? I work here!" I snuck another glance inside. The club was indeed filled with men, dancing and kissing, and some were even naked. A jolt of excitement moved through my body.

"Where am I?" I asked.

"You're in Heaven."

"Heaven?"

"It's a sex club. Now get out of here!" he said as he gently shoved me back toward the stairs.

Later that night, I saw my manager and asked him what that was all about. "Only men?" I said, "And they're allowed to have sex? Who cleans up afterward? There was penis everywhere!"

He just laughed and rolled his eyes.

The next evening when I arrived at work, I noticed the schedule no longer had the letter "D" next to my name, letting me know I was working in the disco. Instead, there was an "H." I had a new job.

I entered Heaven before the music started. Without people, it didn't have the same mystique as the night before. It smelled like stale beer, cheap air freshener, and a certain "something else." The disco itself was small, with a long bar running down the sidewall, which was lined with framed pictures of naked men in bondage. I was the only cisgender woman allowed to enter the club. I was told to serve drinks behind the bar and stay there, unless I had to pee. Then I'd have to leave the club and go downstairs to Limelight and use the one there. I was dying to know what the hell went on in that bathroom that they didn't want me to see or, worse, interrupt!

There were two bright red doors off the main dance floor. In front of each one was a large vat of condoms that the Gay Men's Health Crisis nonprofit delivered each evening, hoping to encourage the men to play safe. Those doors led to back rooms, painted black and lit with purple lighting, where guys would go and have sex. Once the club opened, those doors were off-limits to me. A couple of times I went back there after hours, when the lights were still on, but no patrons were around. I got to see evidence of strange and diverse sexual practices I didn't fully understand. There were glory holes and cat o' nine tails and chains on the walls and a lot of used condoms discarded on the floor. That's when I figured out that the "something else" was a mixture of body odor, ass, and semen. Like most everything, you get used to it.

Heaven was a perfect place to work for a young woman like me. The men who came there loved me but showed no interest in me sexually; in fact, they were often watchful, amused, and protective . . . especially Billy.

Billy was around fifty-eight when I first met him—tall and very dark skinned, with thick hair graying at the temples. He was born in Ohio and raised a Baptist, like his family had been for generations, and he'd married the only woman he'd ever had sex with. They had four children, whom he cherished, and many grandchildren, whom he'd never met. He never met them because, before they were born, he shared a secret he had held for a long time. Billy was gay. Being gay in his small-town Ohio community was not acceptable, nor could it be tolerated; as a result, he was ostracized by his church and rejected by his family. Billy left Ohio and moved to New York City so he could live out the rest of his life in his truth. He loved and missed his family, but also understood that they could never reconcile his need to express his homosexuality with their need for him to be a "proper" Christian man, father, and husband.

Billy could be lonely and melancholy at times, but also charming, funny, and so openhearted. He often wore tight red-leather pants, a white tank top, black-leather half gloves, and a silver necklace that had a circle with a triangle in it—the symbol for recovery. He had been sober for many years, was deeply committed to the 12-step program, and talked about it often.

Billy adored me. He would hug and kiss me hello and often show up just to see what I was wearing. He got such a kick out of my style and would sweetly tease me about my hair or makeup choices. The only time he would get serious with me was when we discussed my drinking and drug use.

I didn't think my drug use was a big deal; I certainly didn't do more than most of my friends, but I guess I did start using pretty young. I smoked my first cigarette at eight, began drinking and smoking pot at thirteen, and started doing mescaline and coke at fifteen. I enjoyed drugs . . . a lot. Thankfully, in spite of my best efforts, I never became addicted. But nonetheless, I was definitely open to exploring pretty much any substance I had access to—and working in nightclubs, living next to drug dealers, and dating guys who did drugs gave me plenty of opportunities to indulge.

Most nights Billy and I talked across the bar while I poured drinks: Sex on the Beach, Long Island Ice Teas, Jägermeister, shot after shot of tequila. Sometimes someone would come along and chat Billy up, and he'd wink knowingly at me and disappear into the back room, only to reemerge with a smile on his face and a story to tell. After a while, though, I noticed he went into the rooms less and less often. He seemed to prefer sitting at the bar, nursing tonic water on ice, watching the crowd, seeing friends, and talking to me.

Then, for about three weeks, Billy didn't show up at all. I was worried, but I had no way of contacting him—I didn't have his phone number, nor did I have a clue where he lived. I asked a couple of the men at the club; no one seemed to know where he was or what was up. Or, if they did, they weren't saying.

Finally, one evening Billy walks into the club. From what I can tell through the smoke and dim lights, his body looks thinner, almost frail. We make eye contact, and he smiles, waves, and crosses the dance floor toward the bar. I am so relieved to see him that I practically leap over the bar to throw my arms around him. As I do, I notice visible, open sores on his neck and shoulders, dark and scabby. He has one on his cheek, another near his eye. I instinctively pull away.

"Billy, what the hell's on your neck?"

Billy puts his hand to his shoulder, touching one of the sores, and says quietly, "They are symptomatic of my disease."

"What disease?" My heart is beating fast, afraid of the answer.

"AIDS," he says, never once taking his eyes off mine. "I have AIDS."

This is the late 1980s, the height of the AIDS epidemic, with around forty thousand cases reported (there are forty million today). The world has stigmatized the disease and those most affected—especially gay men. Even though I work in a gay sex club and understand that gay men are most likely to become infected, I'm still ignorant about the facts and afraid of contracting the disease myself. As a result, the minute Billy says the word "AIDS," I physically recoil. It happens so fast, and I immediately feel ashamed. I hope Billy hasn't noticed, but of course he has.

A look of hurt and resignation passes over his face as he lowers his eyes and takes a deep breath. I reach out and touch his arm. I know I'm not the first to react that way, and sadly, I won't be the last.

"I'm so sorry," I say. "I just don't . . . I can't . . . I mean, what, how . . . ?" I have no words. No way of knowing what to ask. So I stop talking and take his hands in mine.

Billy studies my face for a moment and then asks, "Do you want to understand more about my disease, Seane?"

"Of course."

Billy explains how he may have contracted it. It was either years of having unsafe sex or during the time he was sharing needles with other people. It could have been any number of moments, any number of men, he says. He goes on to explain what he thinks are the ways someone can get AIDS and the ways they can't. I ask if I could get AIDS if he sweated on me, or kissed me, or if he cried on my shoulder. He answers as many of my questions as he can and readily admits there are things he still doesn't understand. He no longer goes into the back rooms because he doesn't want to risk infecting anyone else. And anyway, he says, most of the men already know he has AIDS and want nothing to do with him in that way. I ask him if there's a cure. He shakes his head no.

Finally, my eyes filling with tears, I ask the question I have to ask, even though I already know the answer.

"Billy, what's going to happen to you?"

Billy smiles sadly, and I can see his gums. They look raw and bloody; his once-white teeth have turned to gray.

"I'm going to die."

Just like that. "I'm going to die."

"Aren't you scared?"

"No," he says, shaking his head, "I'm sad but not scared. Not even a little bit."

"Why?"

"Because of my belief in God."

God? What's that got to do with anything?

I was born in 1966 into an interfaith household. My father was raised Catholic, but his father was Jewish. My mother grew up in a rigid Jewish household. There was a lot of resistance to my parents being together, and it mostly had to do with religion.

When my mother got pregnant at seventeen, my father's mother offered him a Cadillac if he could convince my mother to have an abortion (when my brothers and I were young, my father would often joke that he should've taken the friggin' car!). Because of all the hypocrisy they experienced in the name of religion, my parents decided to raise my brothers and me without any religion at all. We celebrated every gift-giving holiday and even sometimes put a Jewish star on top of the Christmas tree. My father said that if anyone cared to ask, we should tell them that we were agnostic. I didn't quite understand what that meant. If there was a God, my parents would say, it was a loving God. Nonetheless, I picked up enough God-fearing from my Christian friends, their parents, and people at school to figure out that this paternal omnipresent force was watchful, judgmental, and punishing. I became afraid of this unseen entity, which loomed large in the lives of so many, and decided that if this fear and anxiety were what being in relationship with God was all about, I wasn't having it.

At the young age of sixteen, I declared that I was an atheist.

So, when Billy says he isn't afraid to die because of his faith in God, I recoil again.

This time, however, Billy laughs. "Seane, don't you believe in God?"

"No, not at all."

"Tell me why."

I describe the anxiety I felt growing up—a low-grade buzzing, tingly and tight, under my skin—because I thought I was bad. How I used to believe that God would punish me for the choices I made. Choices that might be unconventional, wrong, or naughty. I recount how I used to panic because I was convinced that the people I loved, especially my mom, would be taken away from me if I wasn't "pure" enough—whatever that meant—in my thoughts, words, or deeds. I tell him about the rituals I used to do to stop the anxiety—the counting and touching and repeating things in even numbers—how they always made me feel better.

"But now that I'm older, I feel differently," I continue. "I reject the fantasy that there's a puppeteer controlling our actions. I don't want to believe in anything that means I must be perfect in order to be worthy of love. What kind of bullshit God would want that?" If God is all-loving, all-knowing, all-caring, and so concerned about our happiness, I want to know, then why do some people have so much and others so little? Why are people in pain? Why are they suffering? Why are they dying? Why are you dying? You? What did you ever do to deserve this suffering?

Billy lets me talk, waiting while I'm called away to pour another drink, and listening again as I explain why God doesn't exist and why we are all the better for it.

Billy says he understands why believing in God would be so difficult for me. It was once that way for him too. Then he says, "Seane, would you like to see God here? Right now?"

"Now? Here?" I say as I look around the club. "You can't be serious!"

The music is blasting, and the floor pounds with the beat. A mirrored ball hangs in the center, lights bouncing off it in every direction. Men in various states of undress are dancing, grinding, and making out on the dance floor, oblivious to the intense conversation taking place between Billy and me. Surveying the scene, the last place on Earth I could imagine God to inhabit, I laugh and say, "Sure, Billy, show me God!"

Billy then points to Danny the Wonder Pony. Danny's a white guy who comes to the club most nights. He wears a cowboy hat, chaps, boots, a saddle on his back, and nothing else. For a dollar, you can climb on Danny's back and he'll trot around the dance floor while you hit him with a switch. I look over and see Danny throw his head back as some guy rides him and pulls at his hair. They're both laughing, and I hear Danny whinny like a horse. Billy smiles in Danny's direction and says, "God is right there."

Then Billy points to someone we referred to as a cross-dresser—but who, a few decades later, would likely have identified as a transgender woman. Her name is Violet. She's about 6 foot 5 and often wears a light-blue housedress with black sensible shoes, a short gray wig topped with a small cream-colored hat, and veil that covers part of her face. She also wears white-leather kid gloves and carries a sturdy navy pocketbook. Sometimes when Violet pays for her drink, she'll open her bag and pull money from an old gold change purse. She'll press a silver half-dollar coin into my palm, thanking me for her drink. I save all of them. Violet dresses much like my immigrant Polish grandmother, who used to give me silver dollars when I was a little girl. I saved all of those, too. I keep them together.

Billy catches Violet's attention, smiles, waves, and blows her a kiss. She catches it and pulls it to her heart. Then he turns to me and says, "God is right there."

Then Billy gestures toward two men sitting across from one another at a nearby booth. They're wearing suits and ties and arguing playfully over a pitcher of beer. They look so similar to my very straight, conservative brothers, who would never set foot in a place like Heaven. "God is right there, too."

Billy takes his hand and places it over my heart. He then picks up my hand off the bar where it's been resting and lays it over his own heart, keeping his hand gently pressing upon mine. We look into each other's eyes for a long time. "Seane, God is right here," Billy says, as we firmly press our hands against our hearts. "I'm going to tell you something right now. Something I hope you will remember your whole life . . ." And then he pauses.

"Ignore the story and see the soul. And remember to love. You will never regret it."

He holds my gaze for another moment, then continues. "Danny, Violet, all these people here, you and me . . . it's all a story; it's not who we really are. We are pure love, but we think we're something else. The truth is, we're on a journey to awaken to what that love is, and that journey looks different for everyone. And what is this love we awaken to? It's God, Seane. It's inside us, and it's what connects us to one another. Fully. We just need to wake up out of the crazy dream we're all in and remember who we really are. Not these stories, I'll tell you that. They are a part of our experience, but they are not who we are." With that, Billy turns his head and looks around the room. "Not even close." When he looks back at me, tears are in his eyes.

"Seane," Billy says more solemnly, "we all have karma to burn and lessons to learn and all of it—every experience, every moment, no matter how strange, no matter how dark, no matter how hard, no matter how painful, no matter how funky—is purposeful and will bring us closer to the truth of our essence, to that love. To God. That is why I am not afraid to die. AIDS is just my story; it's not who I am. Doesn't mean I don't feel sad; it just means I can't change what is. That's life. I can learn to love better though. Not in spite of this disease but because of what it can teach me. I can change my perceptions, and in changing the way I see things, perhaps I can grow. This growth can only make me more compassionate, more forgiving, more loving, and more connected. So, was it all bad?"

Billy shakes his head slowly, a small smile on his face, and he continues. "That's what we're all doing, just working it out, living life, and doing the best we can. We're remembering who we really are, and when we do, we will also remember who we are to each other. So, ignore the story and see the soul, Seane. All of us, in our own way, in our own time, are opening to love and will come home to know the God within . . . and the God within all. See the soul," Billy presses his hand more firmly against my heart, "and you will understand what unites us. Look around you Seane."

I turn to look back into the club. Danny's still trotting about, Violet's adjusting her wig, and all the people in Heaven are laughing, dancing, and living their lives, perfectly, in that moment.

"We'll all get to the same place, but in a timeline that is unique to each being. So, take this with you: know that every person is a teacher and every experience a teaching, and that there are angels everywhere guiding us, reminding us, and helping us return home. And when we do come home—and we will—we will know ourselves, we will know each other, and we will know peace."

▼

Billy died about three weeks later.

Over the years, I have sat at the feet of saints and sages, I have traveled to meet beloved teachers and guides, but never have I awakened to the sweet and simple truth of seeing the God within the way I did that night, through the eyes of an angel, my angel, in a place called Heaven.

TEACHINGS FROM HEAVEN
YOGA, CONNECTION, AND LOVE

Although Billy never taught me to twist my body into shapes, breathe deeply, or chant a mantra, he was my first true yoga teacher.

Heaven was hardly a place to do yoga, although I certainly saw a few legs wrapped around heads! What I learned from Billy though went much deeper than the physical practice I was already curious about. He taught me the true meaning of yoga—and how to apply it in my own life—in ways I could never have imagined. Billy knew intuitively what yoga masters have taught for millennia: everything is connected—male-female, heaven-earth, mind-body, matter-consciousness, you and I—and our purpose is to see, feel, celebrate, and be in alignment with that connection and to love the whole of this experience and each other, fully, as it is and as we are.

The themes of interconnectedness, loving-kindness, and mindful actions run all through ancient yogic texts, such as the Upanishads, the Bhagavad Gita, the Hatha Yoga Pradipika, and the Yoga Sutras of Patanjali. Although each of these texts and others mention the *yamas* and the *niyamas*—ways in which we can live more consciously and with greater compassion—the description of these practices in the Yoga Sutras is probably the most well-known to Westerners. The *yamas* is a Sanskrit word that's often translated as "restraints" or "thou shalt nots"; the *niyamas* as "disciplines" or "thou shalts." The yamas focus on the relationship we have with the external world; the niyamas on the relationship we have with ourselves. I'll talk more about these along the way, but I want to focus on the one I think encompasses what Billy was saying most of all: *ahimsa*, which most people know as "do no harm." But it's so much more than that.

FROM SEPARATION TO CONNECTION

The first and most important teaching of yoga, ahimsa, goes beyond the obvious reminder not to kill or physically harm another being. At its deepest level, ahimsa helps us move from separation to connection by seeing the Divine in all things, including ourselves, and being able to connect lovingly and purposefully through that shared divinity. Practicing ahimsa means extending friendliness, compassion, and sympathetic joy to others and, in doing so, offering ourselves the same gifts.

Billy said that we are, first and foremost, pure love, and that God is within each of us. But to *be* love, we must see the beauty inherent in others, even—no, especially—those we struggle to understand. We cannot really know ourselves and we cannot truly love ourselves when we set up barriers that keep us separate from others and allow us to judge what we fail or refuse to understand. When we judge, we project our fears, shame, and guilt onto others and see them as "other." Yoga says there is no "other" and to think otherwise is to do great harm. Swami Kripalu said when we judge ourselves, we break our own hearts. Billy suggested that when we judge others, we disconnect not only from those we judge but from our highest Self—the God within. This, he said, is why there is so much conflict in the world and why peace is so elusive.

As long as we create separation, we will never be free.

Yoga teaches us we are One, that everything is united, which is true, but Billy cautioned me that "being One" does not mean "being the same." Yes, we are all on a journey to awaken and understand the depths of our true nature, but the path we take to get there (the how, when, and where) and the experiences we have along the way are unique to each individual soul.

When you commit to the journey, your work is to pay attention to the process itself and not become fixated on the finish line; to cultivate the skills you need to be present to each moment, no matter how messy, confusing, or irrelevant you think it is; to forgive your stumbling, imperfect humanity; and to vow not to judge someone else for the journey they are on, one you can't possibly understand.

Billy showed me that God, or love, is a constant, unwavering presence in each soul. It is our true essence. The only thing that blocks us from fully embracing the power of this energy is the attachment we have to our smaller self, our ego. Our anger, shame, fear, insecurity, guilt, and grief—our shadow self—can block our light and cloud our understanding. Make no mistake, though, Billy wanted me to know, the light is always there—our work is to expose it, by first uncovering the limiting beliefs that diminish its illumination.

IGNORE THE STORY, SEE THE SOUL

In order to know the God within, you must inhabit every part of yourself, especially the wounded, sad, or injured parts. You must investigate and recognize those shadow parts as well as the light because truth and love dwell in equal measure in both places. If there are aspects of yourself you can't accept, it'll be near impossible to accept the same qualities in others. By learning to love fully your own humanity and journey—seeing it all as holy—you can learn to connect, in love, with the souls around you. Love, Billy said, is the only thing that matters, and we are all connected by this love. This, I would come to understand, is yoga. This, I would come to understand, is God.

As Billy had looked around the club—hardly a bastion of holiness—he wanted me to know that God was in every corner, at every table, and in every person there. But to experience God right then, right there, I needed to "ignore the story and see the soul." I needed to look at Danny, prancing like a pony—a half-naked one, at that—with a guy on his back urging him on, and not make up a story about what brought him to Heaven in the first place or why he was the way he was. Those details shouldn't matter to *me*. That's Danny's deal. Billy wasn't saying I had to jump on Danny's back in order to understand him; he wasn't even saying I had to get on board with what he was doing. To ignore the story means to wipe clean the slate of preconceived judgments; to see God in Danny is to meet him soul-to-soul. To see the soul is to see and feel another person's pain, as well as their joy, their spirit, and their capacity to love. That is the true teaching of yoga, of ahimsa—see the soul and don't sweat the details.

Everyone has a story to tell. We all have well-worn narratives we polish and feed—stories we define ourselves by, stories we trot out to highlight our best selves or defend our worst behaviors. These stories are based on our upbringing, experiences, traumas, fears, karma, curiosities, joys, and losses. In telling me to "ignore the story," Billy wasn't saying I should deny, suppress, or minimize my own story. He wasn't telling me my story didn't have value. He was telling me not to define or limit myself by the stories I choose to tell—and, equally important, not to define or limit others by theirs.

Our stories are important, he wanted me to know, and need to be told. It is how we learn, heal, and empathize. This is especially true for folks who have been historically marginalized. But as Billy suggested, we shouldn't let a single story be the whole story. Look beyond the stories, look beyond your own judgments and prejudices, and see the person fully.

All of our stories—not just the ones we cherry-pick—will guide us to the truth and lead us back home to our authentic light, but they are not the truth itself. The truth comes when we stop identifying with these narratives as absolutes and open to what they have to teach us. And as a result, love bigger and better than we ever thought possible.

Everyone, Billy explained, is ultimately doing the best they can, with what little they know, based on the life they've had, the traumas they've experienced, and the tools they can access for transformation. *All* of it—every experience, every moment—will ultimately allow us to see our attachments and illusions. If we are patient and commit to the inner work,

we can surrender the limitations of our stories, bear witness to the attachment we have to our shadow self, and reframe the narratives in a way that empowers. Doing so will bring us closer to the truth of our essence, to our love.

AIDS was just an aspect of Billy's experience the same way being black, male, gay, a father, or a Baptist was—a part of the journey he was on to open to love—but it didn't define him. That doesn't mean he didn't feel sad or angry or scared about his disease or about any of the losses he had experienced in life. It just means that life *happens*. He couldn't change what is, but he could learn to heal, accept, and forgive, not "in spite of this disease, but because of what it can teach." He couldn't change his story, but he could change his relationship to it, and in doing so, learn something essential and grow. This growth would only make him more compassionate, loving, and connected to himself and the world around him. Which it did. Billy wanted me to understand that he would die with gratitude in his heart because his journey was perfect; it guided him to know love and open to God in ways he could've never imagined.

Remember to love. Everything, everyone, yourself, the world around you.

That is the work. Because if you can be with that love, embrace it, own it, and let it influence all the ways you are in the world, then you will know God, you will be home, and peace in every way possible will be your contribution to this life.

ANGELS ARE EVERYWHERE

Lastly, Billy also helped me understand that we are all each other's teacher, and that angels reveal themselves in curious ways. Make no mistake, your angels are everywhere, waking you up to who you really are. Sometimes teachers will reveal themselves in loving and tender ways; sometimes the teachings will be fierce. Sometimes your teachers will be subtle in their offerings; sometimes they will break your heart. Often the lessons will be incomprehensible; always they will be potent and necessary for the evolution of your soul.

Over the years, I have had many angels guiding me. We all have. Moments happen that add color, texture, and grout to our understanding and move us along the path as we respond to God's call. Nothing is incidental or accidental. Everything, even the hard parts, are essential. Billy showed up at a time in my life and in a way that made it possible for me to receive these lessons. He planted a seed and sent me forward on my path. Lord knows my awakening wasn't going to happen in a conventional church or temple! I had too much resistance to hear any other message beside separation and exclusivity, something I already felt within myself. Instead, the message of acceptance, forgiveness, and love—as God's truest expression—spoke authentically to my heart and left an indelible imprint upon it.

It would take years though, and many angels, for me to understand and embody all that Billy shared with me that night. This book is that journey. These are my stories and the teachings they uncovered to help me understand the interconnection we all share and our responsibility to be of service to that connection for the good of all.

What makes us who we are in this moment is the path we take, a path with no particular destination or endpoint. Each step forward or backward informs and determines the quality of our evolving soul. It adds depth to our experience, but still, it is not who we are; it's just the journey we take to come home—only to find we've never left, and what we've been looking for has been within us all along.

WAKING UP AT LIFE CAFÉ

2

MANHATTAN IN THE MID-1980s was remarkable. These were the final days of the gritty, dirty, and dangerous New York before corporatization and gentrification took over. Times Square was still rows and rows of porn theaters and strip clubs; West 14th Street was where meat was butchered and sold, the streets shiny from grease and blood; prostitutes worked 9th Avenue just outside the Lincoln Tunnel; and the Christodora House on Avenue B, where my grandparents used to socialize when they were young, had not yet turned into high-priced condos.

Even before I landed in Heaven, I got a day job waiting tables at Life Café. The café, a small corner shop on 10th Street and Avenue B, had a tin ceiling, uneven black-and-white tile floors, and a step in the middle of the restaurant, which someone would inevitably trip over at least once a day. David Life was the owner, Sharon Gannon the head waitress, and Eddie Stern, the delivery guy. The walls were covered in artwork, mostly created by David, who was already considered the grandfather of the East Village art scene—I think he was thirty-four years old at the time. He was tall, thin, with bleached-blonde hair to his shoulders, and looked like a handsome Iggy Pop with tattoos, skin-tight jeans, and black high-tops.

Sharon was a performance-art priestess. An artist of life. She was gorgeous and alert. You didn't mess with Sharon. She was smarter than everyone in the room and demanded excellence, even if it was just the precise way you lined up the ketchups at the end of your shift. She would walk through the café focused and ready to work, wearing fishnets, a leopard-print bodysuit, and a tutu. It's hard to be intimidated by someone in a tutu, but I most certainly was!

Eddie was a soft-spoken man, quiet but watchful, with long hair that hung down to his butt. He was easy to be around, thoughtful and kind toward everyone; when we did have a chance to talk, his dry wit cracked me up. He rode a bright-red bicycle with a metal basket box in front with a lock on it to keep the food from being stolen.

On my very first day at Life, a customer came in, a young woman in her early twenties. She sat down in my section, asked politely for water, a cup of coffee, and the bathroom key. I delivered her requests and then waited for her to come out so I could take the rest of her order. After about fifteen minutes, I asked my manager, Sadik, if he thought everything was all right. "Your customer, your problem," he said, and handed me another bathroom key. I knocked on the bathroom door and asked if she was okay. Nothing. I knocked again. No response. Finally, I used the key to open the door, but it wouldn't budge. I pushed a little harder, creating just enough space to get my head in. I saw the young woman lying on the floor next to the toilet, her feet pressed up against the door. She was naked from the waist down, her pants around her calves. She had a syringe needle sticking out of the inside of her left elbow. There was blood pooled around the entry point of the needle, the dark red trickle snaking down her arm and onto the floor. Her eyes were slightly open and watery; there was a pale, foamy substance bubbling from her mouth. I ran and called 911. The police had to break down the door to get her out. It wasn't the last time I saw an overdose or a dead body at Life Café.

Life attracted a broad and diverse population of people. I waited on Allen Ginsberg and William Burroughs, serving them for years before I knew who they were. They always sat in my section drinking free refills of coffee and bantering back and forth—for hours. I waited on Cher, Matt Dillon, punk-rocker Richard Hell, famous artists and writers, politicians, homeless people, squatters, and drug addicts, often all at the same time. Curtis Sliwa and the Guardian Angels, community vigilantes who volunteered to keep the peace, roamed Alphabet City in their red berets. They broke up many a fight at the café, including one started by my then-boyfriend, Michael, when a customer, who was drunk, pushed me and then lifted his hand to slap my face. I swear Michael flew over the tables and sucker-punched the guy before his hand could make contact with my cheek. All hell broke loose, tables turning, dishes crashing. Suddenly, the Guardian Angels appeared. They stepped in and stopped the violence before it escalated any further.

Pretty much everyone on staff was doing drugs, including me. We used to cut lines of coke on the tank of the toilet, cover it with a bowl, and one-by-one take turns snorting a line right off the filthy porcelain, or we'd go into the back garden and smoke cocaine out of a menthol cigarette, listening for the kitchen bell that told us our order was ready. Smoking coke was my favorite way to get high. I loved the minty taste against the sharp, ashy, acidic burn of tobacco and coke. Many nights, the barman, Jim, who was just getting hooked on heroin, would make coffee drinks and pour beer, while simultaneously vomiting into a nearby garbage can. It was an interesting time, to say the least.

David, Sharon, and Eddie were all into yoga, even then. Tara Rose, a young dancer in the East Village, was teaching yoga at her apartment, and Sharon would often go there to take class. I'd overhear Sharon talking about the benefits of the practice and what a wonderful "yogini" Tara was. I'd sometimes see Tara, all young, white, and pretty, in high-waisted jeans, a rock-and-roll T-shirt, and Candies wedge shoes clumping in earnest down 10th Street, and then reflect on the images of yoga that I had in my head. *That's not what a yoga person looks like.*

Of course, I really didn't know what a yoga person was supposed to look like. I had seen bejeweled Indian gods and goddesses painted blue, straddling tigers, or holding up the severed heads of demons. Were they yogis? What about the stoned-out, dreadlocked hippies who gathered on the lawn in Central Park twisting themselves into pretzel shapes? I suppose they considered themselves yogis too. All I knew was that yoga came out of a religious tradition, just like Judaism and Catholicism, and I had no interest in participating in anything that had to do with any kind of God—and certainly not multiple gods!

Between serving up mega-burritos and stir-fried veggies, I picked up bits and pieces of conversations about yoga and alternative health practices. Sharon, David, Eddie, and Tara were cool and hip, creative and smart; I couldn't reconcile my preconceptions of spiritual practice with the actions and beliefs of these people, whom I admired. Once I was pretty sure I couldn't be "converted," I started to pay a little more attention to their conversations and grew more curious. Not that I was completely swayed, though. I do remember once Sharon talking about the health benefits of a coffee enema. I was way too embarrassed to ask how it worked and instead stared at my latte and wondered how the hell you'd get that up your ass and why anyone would want to. It was all so foreign to me. In all fairness, I was fresh off the NJ Transit 197 bus. Where I grew up, you got vaccinated, took your antibiotics, and pretty much followed the instructions of your allopathic doctor without question.

David didn't favor one class of people over another and was loathe to throw anyone out, no matter who they were or how they behaved. I'm pretty sure he lost a small fortune giving away food and coffee each day. But that didn't matter to him. In his mind, all people deserve respect, food to eat, and a place of sanctuary, even at the expense of his own business. David was incredibly generous, but it kind of sucked if you were working on the days he was there. He had no problem letting people hang out all day, play chess, and nurse free refills. If they didn't have any money for food, he would make sure they got a bowl of rice with tahini sauce and a cup of coffee on the house. If you complained that they were taking up tables, David would shoot you a look of disappointment that made you feel like such an asshole for focusing on the few bucks you would have earned. But truthfully? Those few bucks didn't matter since we were all skimming money off the top anyway and pocketing it (sorry David!). It all balanced out in the end.

▼

About a year into my time there, Sharon and David went to India to study with Swami Nirmalananda, a beloved and well-respected Indian guru. When they got back, the change in David was particularly apparent. He'd always had a compassionate and accepting nature, a gentleness that made me want to be more like him. When he came back from India, all of his positive qualities seemed magnified, and all of my negative qualities stood out in stark contrast—in my mind anyway. I was young, anxious, and insecure. I wanted so much to be accepted by others, yet I didn't know how. I tried too hard, laughed too loud, and did everything I could to both fit in and rebel. But inwardly I was aching to relax, and as my mom would tell me . . . just *be*. David, on the other hand, had a very calming effect on everyone around him; he seemed so secure in who he was. I wanted that.

When David and Sharon came back from India that first time, David wanted real change at the café. I didn't blame him. On some level, I knew that things had gotten fairly out of control and the environment was becoming unhealthy. Like I said, we were all stealing from the cash box. Everything was written on check pads, so it was easy to alter the check after someone paid their bill and slide the extra cash into your apron pocket. I was already a pro at this. I had fudged receipts at Krauszer's convenience store in Jersey, when I was still in high school, to get the money to move to New York in the first place. I felt no guilt or shame about stealing; after all, I was working "so hard," and the minimum wage and meager tips I earned didn't match the effort I put in. I felt entitled to it. At Life, most of us were in collusion anyway, so no one was eager to point out how wrong we were.

Then David started to clean house. He let a lot of people go, including those who were obviously abusing drugs. He basically told us that we could keep doing drugs, but we'd have to find a new job. Or, we could clean up our act, stay at Life, and learn a thing or two about living more "consciously." Essentially, David was inviting us all to practice yoga and live by its principles, which had little to do with stepping onto a mat and everything to do with developing our awareness.

For example, one of the first things David did was change the menu to include more vegan options to reflect his and Sharon's commitment to animal rights, which they spoke passionately about. I knew that he wanted to create a healthier environment for us all, but I didn't understand veganism at all. I was raised a meat eater and never really gave much thought to the fact that my hamburger was actually cow flesh, or that the "nuggets" were chicken, or that my bacon was actually pig. It just tasted good.

All I knew was that David was eliminating some of my favorite meals at the café, and I was annoyed. Why was he imposing his views and diet on everyone else? How was I supposed to get my protein without my chicken chimichangas?

One afternoon, a couple weeks later, I was at my friend's apartment on 14th Street, and I saw a book on his coffee table called *In the American West*, by Richard Avedon. I lazily flipped through the pages, looking at the beautiful black-and-white portraits of Midwestern working-class folks. And then I saw it. A photo of a man in overalls staring back at me. He had taken the freshly severed head of a cow, blood dripping from its neck, eyes open, tongue lolling out, and placed it over his own head like a mask. This man worked in a factory farm; slaughtering animals was his job. For the first time in my life, I saw real pain and suffering in an animal's eyes. If I couldn't imagine someone slaughtering a living, breathing human, how could I possibly be okay with someone killing an animal? An animal who feels and connects, grieves and loves? That was it for me. Seeing that image reinforced all that David and Sharon had been saying about animal abuse and the horrors of factory farms. I never touched red meat again.

Another lesson in self-awareness came my way after I had worked there a couple years. Here's how it all went down.

▼

David pairs me with a young woman whom he's hired to bus tables. Her other job is dancing naked on stage for the punk rock band the Butthole Surfers. She's very young, does a lot of drugs, is socially awkward, and is slow to learn. She epitomizes the kind of people David often hires—people he feels sorry for or concerned about. Whether they actually have skills to do the job rarely enters into the equation.

I can't stand working with her. She often seems high and will lazily swipe at my tables with a cloth, essentially smearing food across the table or brushing it onto the floor for someone to step on. Sometimes I catch her just staring off into space. One day David overhears me giving her shit. I've just watched her drop a plate on the floor, where it shatters into pieces, food splattering everywhere, including all over my boots. I glare at her. She looks up at me pitifully, but before she can say anything, I stomp away, look back over my shoulder, and say, "You fucking idiot!" David pulls me aside.

"Why did you say that to her?"

I bend down and wipe some ketchup off my leg and say, "Because she is an idiot. She doesn't know what she's doing. She can't even bus a table right! David, seriously. She should be fired."

I'm sure he'll appreciate how conscientious I am.

He doesn't. He gently but firmly puts me in my place. "Seane, it may not always feel like it, but things will come easier for you than they will for other people. It's hardly fair, but it's just the way it is. It's called privilege. Some have it and some don't. You do. And because you do, you also have a responsibility to be much more compassionate and understanding to those who may not get the opportunities you'll get in this life. So be nice. Go out of your way to support her. Go out of your way to understand her. Don't add to the challenges she may already have. Be patient. You don't need to know where she's come from or what her story is. You just need to be kind."

I get the compassion part, but privilege? How is it possible that someone like me has privilege? I'm a kid, for fuck's sake, and an uneducated one at that. I have no money and work as a waitress. It would take years before I would understand what it was he was teaching me and what it had to do with yoga. Meanwhile, I'm about to get another lesson in yoga from a most unlikely source: a hard-core punk band.

Stephan, the lead singer of the False Prophets, comes into Life Café often. He wears a Nazi-like mustache with handlebars and has long nails painted black that curl and twist many inches from his hand. He also carries a walking stick with some kind of skull on it. But honestly, he looks more menacing than he is. Whenever he comes into the café, he's always friendly. It amuses me to watch him try to maneuver a fork around those four-inch nails.

One day, Stephan sits down in my section, orders a coffee, and we casually chat as usual. Then, out of the blue, he asks me if I would perform on stage with the band at CBGB's, a loud, raucous downtown rock-and-roll club that famously hosts bands like Blondie, the Ramones, Talking Heads, The Police, and Television.

He tells me he'll pay me a hundred bucks if I get up on the stage with the band and stand absolutely still. No matter what the band or the audience does (and he promises me I won't be touched or get hurt), I am not to smile or react—or even blink if I can help it. I'm to stare straight ahead and then, over the course of an hour, move my head ever so slightly until I'm staring off to the left. The trick is to not allow anyone to see my head move. Of course I say yes.

At the show, the crowd is wild. There's a mosh pit in the center, and, as the band starts playing, noise and chaos engulf me. Although I can *feel* the band jumping and hear them screaming, I can't actually see what they're doing. I can only see the audience in front of me and they're raging to the music.

I turn all of my attention to a single point in front of me. No matter what's happening, I never take my eyes off that particular spot. I focus on my breathing, extending each exhalation as long as I can, which helps me feel calm in the center of all the noise and commotion. Whenever the time seems right, I move my head a fraction of an inch, shifting my gaze as I do.

Soon the chaos blurs in front of me, becoming something I can be part of and yet separate from. I feel calm and steady on my feet and utterly present. I don't think about anything else, my gaze stays single pointed, my breath deep, and even when the crowd screams at me or the band gets too close to my body, I never flinch. Afterward I feel strangely grounded, even though I had been in the center of a whirlwind.

Although I had no way of knowing it at the time, I was actually doing yoga. Not *asana*—the physical poses associated with yoga—not yet. But other limbs the ancient texts present as integral to the yoga path: *pranayama* (controlling and extending the breath), *pratyahara* (withdrawing the senses), and *dharana* (one-pointed concentration). These practices certainly became central to my practice later in my life, but seriously? I could never have imagined I'd be introduced to them like this. The evolution of the soul can be really weird like that.

TEACHINGS FROM LIFE
AWAKENING, DISCOVERY, AND THE YAMAS

Sharon, David, and Eddie were fiercely committed to yoga. All you had to do was pay attention to their conversations, and you'd pick up interesting tidbits about this sacred spiritual practice. So that's what I did. I would linger at the bar or take my time wiping down the tables near where they were chatting and listen. What I really noticed was that yoga had become a way of life for David and Sharon, especially after they returned from India. They had changed—not physically so much as in their attitude—in ways that made me want to be more like them. The kindness, compassion, and thoughtfulness they exhibited made me feel at ease in their presence. I wanted to feel at ease all the time, especially in my own skin, but I rarely did, so I thought maybe they had a "trick" or two up their sleeve that would help me.

At the time, I didn't think the lessons I was learning had anything to do with yoga. But looking back, I can see that David and Sharon exemplified the core of the yogic teachings: always be kind because when one being suffers, we all suffer. As far as I knew, yoga was a religious practice from India and seemed to have something to do with contorting your body into odd poses and chanting OM. I would come to find out that, although the poses were the most recognized aspect of the practice in the West, they were actually only a small piece of what yoga is really all about. So how was what I was learning yoga teachings?

Let's start with the definition of yoga. *Yoga* means to "yoke" or "to join together and make whole." (It comes from the Sanskrit root *yuj*, which means "to join or unite.") That doesn't mean you corral the "bad" parts of yourself to make sure they don't mess things up for the "good" parts. To join together and make whole is to welcome and begin to accept *all* aspects of yourself, to notice the good, the not-so-good, and the truly cringe-worthy. *Yoking* also means connecting your individual soul with the Divine, Cosmic Consciousness, God, or whatever else you call this transcendent state of awareness. And, as Billy expressed, to remember that there is no separation between your soul and the Divine, between yourself and others, or between all of us and the planet.

Yoga harkens back thousands of years, showing up in rock carvings of yogis sitting in lotus position and in texts such as the Vedas (the oldest known scriptures of Hinduism). And yet it has so much to teach us today. The Yoga Sutras, compiled around 200 CE by a historical, perhaps mythical, figure named Patanjali, is probably the most well-known of yoga's venerable texts—at least in the West. In it, Patanjali presents the Eight Limbs of Yoga: guidelines for how we can live a happier, healthier, less reactive, and more loving life and how we can liberate ourselves and others from suffering.

As a philosophy, yoga asks us to begin with what is most tangible: our relationships to others and to ourselves. And then we move on, diving deeper toward the core of our being, our Divine essence. So, we start with the yamas, or ethical restraints, the first of the eight limbs, which offer five ways to pay more loving attention to our environment. The yamas invite us to notice how our actions affect not only others but ourselves. We all know the Judeo-Christian Golden Rule, "Do unto others as you would have them do unto you." The yamas show us how to practice it.

The second limb, the niyamas, or observances, offers five daily practices to help strengthen our connection to ourselves; it invites us to clean up our act to make space for liberation to happen. It requires a willingness to reflect on who we are and the attachments we have to our own stories. Once we commit to the yamas and niyamas, Patanjali says, we can then move on to the other limbs of yoga by preparing the physical body through asana, extending and controlling the breath using pranayama, moving the senses inward with *pratyahara*, cultivating the power of concentration through *dharana*, meditating on the Divine (*dhyana*), and finally, entering into union with the Divine, a process called *samadhi*. The entire journey brings us back home to our true nature.

Of course, when I first started working at Heaven and Life Café, I hadn't even done a yoga pose and didn't have a clue what a yoga sutra was. But I had been shown the power of the yamas through my relationships with Billy and David Life. So, let's dissect the yamas from the point of view of our everyday lives—and the multitude of kindnesses we witness along the way.

It would take me getting on an actual yoga mat before the niyamas and the other six limbs would begin to reveal themselves in a way I could understand.

AHIMSA (NON-HARMING)

The five ethical restraints begin with ahimsa, which is pretty much all you need to remember: Do. No. Harm. Always. Be. Kind. I got my first come-to-ahimsa lesson when David changed the menu to include a lot more vegan options. That demonstrated their commitment to animal rights, which influenced my own decision to become first a vegetarian and then a vegan. I got my second lesson when he called me out for being mean to my coworker. I thought that by chewing her out, David would see that I was responsible, and he would like or respect me more. By taking her down, I could lift myself up and be seen as hardworking, loyal, and trustworthy, qualities that made me feel more valued and lovable. Instead, David showed me how I used my privilege and what little power I had to create separation, and how that caused unnecessary pain.

In truth, I was not only harming my coworker, I was hurting myself. I felt I had to look, act, and be a certain way in order for people to love me. This is called ego—the ways in which we identify ourselves and declare to ourselves and the world around us: "This is who I am." After all, who am I when I'm not those things? Am I still valuable? Am I still lovable? Practicing ahimsa helps us trust that what makes us valued as a soul isn't about how we look or what we accomplish, but how we treat others and how we honor ourselves.

Although ahimsa is most often translated as non-harming, it really means much more than that. It means love. Not the squishy, touchy-feely type of love generally associated with romantic sentiments, but love as a primordial force that sustains, uplifts, and connects all souls to one another. Mahatma Gandhi, the Indian activist who coined the English translation "non-harming," later regretted it because, he said, it focused on the negative. Instead, he suggested we think of ahimsa as "a force which is more positive than electricity" and that we see this all-pervasive force as the ultimate truth.

There's a reason that ahimsa is the first "commandment" of yoga. If we don't practice loving-kindness, how can we possibly expect to live in peace with others; how can we possibly feel good about ourselves? Ahimsa also means non-judgment, which is what Billy taught me when he encouraged me to accept others, regardless of where they came from or what their stories were.

In truth, you can't successfully practice the rest of the yamas or niyamas without adhering to the principle of ahimsa, without understanding how your actions and thoughts can either cause suffering or alleviate it.

SATYA (TRUTHFULNESS)

This second yama is associated with truthfulness; it literally means "that which is." Rolf Sovik of the Himalayan Institute says *satya* means "seeing and reporting things as they are rather than the way we would like them to be." Basically, this yama encourages you to be truthful, to stay open to hearing the truth, and to only tell the truth if you can tell it with clarity, kindness, and compassion—in other words, ahimsa before satya.

Obviously, the whole truth-telling thing wasn't my MO at Life Café or pretty much anywhere else I worked or hung out. I lied in my relationships, and I lied to myself. I had subconsciously crafted a persona I wanted the world to see, one in which I was charming, cute, a little cocky, and doing just fine, thank you very much. I didn't understand back then that the self I had constructed actually kept me separate from others and contributed mightily to the loneliness and anxiety that plagued me from time to time. It took me a long time to see all the ways I was untrue to myself, all the ways I refused to see what was real. Telling the truth, in my mind, meant I would have to admit to feelings, experiences, and actions I wasn't proud of, that made me ashamed, or that would show the world I wasn't truly worthy of anyone's respect or love.

Before you blurt out something you think someone needs to hear—or beat yourself up over something you've done—ask yourself these four questions: *Is it in fact true? Is it necessary? Is it kind? Is it useful?* Although they've been attributed to everyone from Krishna in the Bhagavad Gita to Quakers, and even Krishnamurti, they offer sound advice. Satya asks us to stop lying to ourselves as well, to commit to discovering the truth of who we really are, by gently and tenderly polishing the lens through which we can understand the narratives that live in our bodies. Although that sounds daunting, it's actually easier—and way less stressful—than pretending to be something you're not. In fact, being truthful feels lighter, freer, and, in the end, more liberating.

ASTEYA (NON-STEALING)

On a practical level, *asteya* is an easy one. Don't take anything that doesn't belong to you. Right? I didn't do so well with this yama, either. I repeatedly stole from my employers—all of them—and didn't even feel bad about it. In fact, I felt entitled to those extra "bonuses" because I worked *so hard* and making minimum wage seemed so unfair. Besides, everyone else was doing it too. I stole affection from would-be lovers because I was bored, insecure, anxious, and afraid—without realizing how my actions were harming both me and them.

Of course asteya means not stealing money or objects, but it can also mean not appropriating other people's ideas and calling them your own, not stealing away someone's affections when you have no intention of reciprocating, or even not taking advantage of someone's generosity. So much of this, the wise

old yogis say, happens when you feel insecure, lonely, or fearful. That's when you may try to fill the void by pretending to be someone you're not, hoping to gain the attention and approval of others. You steal from yourself when you minimize your own troubles, shaking them off as no big deal; beat yourself up for thinking you suffer in the first place when so many others are worse off; or when you refuse to be tender and compassionate with yourself. Above all, this yama is about generosity and gratitude, it's about learning to say yes, and it's a reminder that you are enough—that you have everything you need within you.

BRAHMACHARYA (TURNING INWARD)

Most people think of *brahmacharya* as practicing sexual abstinence or, at least, being constant in their relationships, choosing ones that are mutually supportive and move both people toward the highest truth. Oh boy. I pretty much failed at this one too. I was a serial cheater because I craved love and attention and lacked self-confidence (even as I exuded it). So, the only way I knew how to find validation was to turn on the charm and turn up the volume on my sexuality, using my powers of seduction to reaffirm my self-worth.

Luckily, brahmacharya is much more nuanced than sexual continence. The translation I've heard that I love the most is "walking in the presence of God" or "walking in God-consciousness," which means turning inward and not depending on sensual pleasures or outside stimulation to bring you joy. When you act with God-consciousness, you are less likely to make impulsive, self-indulgent decisions that aren't very mindful. Finally, practicing brahmacharya focuses the mind on the task at hand and helps us dedicate our energies to both our inner work and our work in the world.

APARIGRAHA (NON-GRASPING)

The final yama, which means non-grasping or non-possessiveness, is also fairly straightforward. You suffer when you become obsessed with or attached to material goods. When you become possessed by your possessions, when you covet what others have—even things of a spiritual nature—you move further away from the present moment and from realizing your own true essence.

Aparigraha doesn't mean you should sell all your possessions and live a monk's life. But it does mean that you should bring material things into your life consciously, engaging with them in a way that supports your highest values.

Aparigraha can also mean holding on to people in your life, ideas about yourself, false identities, jobs, and other things long past their "expiration" date. That's where I got tripped up. I didn't have a true sense of self yet; therefore, I looked for identification through the persona I created, coveting bits of style and personality from the people around me. This included adopting their phrasing or habits and liking the cigarettes they smoked or brand of coffee they drank. I was young and trying to come into my own but had no idea what that meant. There was never enough of anything though that could make me feel truly whole. No matter if I nailed the perfect outfit or got my hands on something that made me feel interesting or important, it was never enough. I always wanted the next best thing. I also had a really hard time letting go of anything or anyone in my life. Even as a child, when my mother would try to get rid of old toys or stuffed animals—things I hadn't used in a long time—I couldn't bear the loss, and I would liberate them from the trash, apologize to them, and return them to their rightful place.

YOGA IS NOW

The life lessons of kindness and connection I learned from David and Billy made sense to me, but I didn't really equate them with yoga per se. Looking back, what I was learning was that yoga is *now*—the first directive in the Yoga Sutras. Yoga. Is. Now. There is no better time to practice yoga than right this minute, when you are in the middle of your chaotic, mixed-up life. When nothing seems to be going right or when you find the people around you to be deeply irritating or when you're standing in a nightclub with people acting in ways you don't understand or making choices you'd never in a million years make. It's easy to be kind and compassionate and to see the Divine in others when they're nice to you or the same as you. But practicing the precepts (the yamas and niyamas) when people are different? Or assholes? Or when you're an anxious mess and your life is in shambles? Not so much.

Every single moment in life is yoga—every moment, the light and the shadow; every experience, the good and the weird; and every being, those you adore and those you don't. It's all yoga, and it's all purposeful for the evolution of your soul. We think we are separate, but that is the lie that we tell ourselves. We are connected to everything and everyone, just like Billy said. Yoga opens our eyes so we can see clearly who we are and who we are to each other. This awakening gives us permission to be more joyous, connected, understanding, compassionate, and loving, right here, right *now*.

Quite frankly, this is good enough for me. If we can all surrender to the highest aspects of ourselves that yoga encourages, then we can commit to a life well lived—and loved—for the benefit of all.

3

AN UNFAMILIAR FEELING

EVERYWHERE I LOOKED, people were wearing head-to-toe white—long, flowing, wide-legged pants and tunics. Some even carried sandalwood necklaces in their palms, muttering to themselves, eyes closed, as they fingered the individual beads. After hearing about yoga for years and witnessing the changes in David and Sharon, I'd decided to see for myself what the hoopla was about. I'd come to Integral Yoga where everything was so serene and so clean. Except for me. I looked down at my gray sweatpants, grease stains on the thighs from where I had wiped my hands after working on my motorcycle. I was still wearing the oversized Siouxsie and the Banshees T-shirt that I had slept in the night before, but luckily I'd had enough sense to put on a bra before I left the apartment. I hadn't showered and knew without a doubt that black eyeliner and mascara lay smeared under my eyes. It was pretty much how I looked most days, but in that particular environment, I was a bit of a mess.

I entered the Integral store, which doubled as a reception area, walked over to the counter, and was told to sign in and remove my shoes. Everyone was barefoot. I kicked off my black-leather Screaming Mimi combat boots, tossed them toward the rest of the shoes on the floor, but left my socks on. Going barefoot in a public place that wasn't a park or beach kinda grossed me out, plus I often cut and peeled the skin off my big toes and heels when I was anxious and didn't want anyone to see the shredded skin or the Band-Aids. The woman behind the counter, also wearing white, looked calm and sweet. I noticed, when she raised her arm to reach for something, she had a thick patch of armpit hair. Did Sharon shave her pits? I'd have to investigate this. Maybe that was a sign you were a real yogi. Note to self: stop shaving, buy something white and . . . take a bath.

The woman told me that class would start soon, and I should just wait. So I checked out the books on the shelves with titles like *Bhakti Yoga* and *Beauty of Ramayana*. Integral was a Sivananda studio, which meant nothing to me at the time. I just figured all yoga was the same. According to the Vedanta text I was thumbing through, though, there were actually *four* paths of yoga, which meant four different ways to become enlightened. One was strictly devotional (*bhakti*), another centered on knowledge (*jñana*), still another was dedicated to service or action (*karma*), and the fourth (*raja*) focused mainly on meditation. So enlightenment's the goal? Huh. Who knew? I rolled my eyes, snapped the book closed, and put it back on the shelf.

I picked up another book and flipped through it. It was filled with words written in a language I couldn't identify. I glanced back toward the receptionist, remembering the tattoo I had seen on her upper arm, a band of lettering written just like the words in the book. I had no idea I was looking at Sanskrit. Pictures of deities, gods, and goddesses in intriguing and sensual scenes were sprinkled throughout the book. The images were alluring, but my distrust of religion caused me to frown at the pictures, close the book, and return it to the shelf. What the hell was I doing there? I glanced at my boots splayed out awkwardly where I had tossed them. Everyone else's shoes were lined up neatly in a row. I thought, *Well, that just sums up my whole life.* I considered going home.

▼

Just then, the woman behind the desk announces that it's time for class. I stand up and sigh. *Okay, let's do this.* I follow the others up some narrow, creaky stairs and into one of the rooms above. The floors in the room are wooden and uneven, the room itself stark and smelling faintly of BO, mold, and incense. In the front of the room is a small altar with candles and pictures and statues of some of the same Indian gods and goddesses I've just seen in the book I picked up. There's a big fat guy with the head of an elephant sitting down with one foot on a mouse and a woman with many arms riding a tiger. But my favorite is a picture of a woman with wild hair and her tongue out, wearing a necklace of severed heads. She's scary, fierce, and intense looking. Could she really be a goddess? She hardly looks peaceful. A woman walks by me, glances in the direction I'm looking, smiles, and says quietly, "Kali-Ma!" I grin and wrap my own wild and uncombed hair into a topknot. The room feels sacred, purposeful, and a bit strange to my Western sensibilities, and yet I'm oddly comfortable in what appears to be a place of worship. I hang back a little to watch what everyone else is doing; then, following their lead, I grab a mat and what looks like a little pillow, which makes a crunching sound when I squeeze it.

I find a spot toward the back of the room and off to the side where I can observe without anyone noticing me. I roll out my mat, lining it up evenly between the floorboards, place the pillow toward the front, and sit down on it, cross-legged, like everyone else. The other students all sit perfectly still, eyes closed, palms in their lap. I take advantage of their closed eyes to study them and this space, while I wait for the teacher to arrive.

He comes in quietly, an air of importance and reserve about him. I'm pretty sure he's some kind of holy man, like a guru, the kind of person Sharon and David spoke about meeting in India. He doesn't look Indian though. He looks more like an uncle or cousin from the Jewish side of my family. Less like a guru, more like a rabbi. He's white and older, with scraggly gray and white hair hanging loosely past his shoulders and a similarly colored beard. He gathers up his white pants, kneels down, takes his seat in the front of the room, and drapes a white shawl over his shoulders. I smile to myself, thinking he looks more suited to reciting the haftarah than teaching a yoga class. He then picks up a pair of metal discs connected by a leather string and clinks them together three times.

The reverberation alerts the students, causing their spines to straighten and the backs of their heads to lengthen on their necks. I glance at the person closest to me and could see her eyes are still shut. I look to the others and see that their eyes are also still shut. I look at the guru-rabbi. His eyes are open, and he's staring at me, one eyebrow raised. He smiles and makes a gesture with his hands, indicating that I should shut my eyes too. I do.

I've never meditated before. I try to keep my back straight all the while wondering how long we have to stay there. I wonder if I'm doing it right. I wonder if I'm supposed to be thinking. *But if I'm not supposed to be thinking, what am I supposed to be doing instead? Is everyone else thinking too? That can't be right. We can't all be just sitting here thinking. Are they thinking about me, like I'm thinking about them? I wonder what I'm going to eat later and if yoga can help me stop smoking and if my boyfriend really loves me and if maybe I should take the bus home this weekend to see my mom. I miss my mom. I really love my mom. My mom's so cool. It's really hot in here. Maybe it will rain? My nose itches. Am I allowed to scratch my nose? I fidget on the crunchy pillow, my hips aching, my right foot asleep inside my sock. There's no way I'm taking off my socks. Not ever. Maybe I should get a cat . . . ?*

My thoughts go on like that for what seems like an eternity, one tumbling into the next, in no particular order and with no particular point. I start to get panicky, so I open my eyes. The teacher begins to sing, not sing really, but recite words I can't identify in a singsongy, droning kind of way. He finishes a line, and then the rest of the class repeats it back. I just stare ahead. I guess we're chanting? I move my mouth, to make it look like I was too, hoping nothing audible escapes.

Next up, he asks us to breathe, in and out, very fast and deep through the nose. I try, but my whole torso keeps lifting up and down. A light trail of snot escapes out my nose, and I repeatedly wipe at it with the back of my hand while glancing self-consciously around the room. This goes on for quite a while. Periodically I have to stop to cough, the tar from cigarettes reacting to the quick compression of my lungs. And then, after a bit, he tells us to breathe normally and reflect on how we feel. The deep breathing makes me feel dizzy and a bit sick to my stomach. I sit there reflecting on my nausea and reluctantly begin again when he tells us to. *Yoga isn't particularly glamorous,* I think, wiping away more snot and coughing up a lung.

Then he has us close the right side of our nose with our thumb, inhale through the left nostril, close both nostrils, release the thumb, and exhale through the right side—and repeat starting with the right side. Ugh, I'm not getting it. I'm inhaling and exhaling, my thumb and index finger often closing both nostrils at the wrong time, stopping me from breathing altogether. Finally I give up and just fake it, moving my fingers randomly across my nose.

After that, we're invited to lie down on our back. I welcome that and would gratefully stay there all day. Instead, he tells us to come to standing and "find Tadasana." I stand limply at the front of my mat, looking around at everyone else, who appear to be standing at attention, staring forward, tight and rigid. "Feet together, straighten your legs," the teacher commands. "Arms to the side, long spine. Sturdy, like a mountain!" He tells us to feel our feet on the ground beneath us. "Extend your roots deep into the earth, and you will find your strength and refuge there, with the Mother!" *Mother? Whose mother?* I do as I'm told—I think. But, truthfully, I haven't a clue what I'm doing. I don't feel like a mountain. *What the fuck does a mountain even feel like?* Everyone in the room looks so serious in their mountain, so I make myself look serious too and stare straight ahead without blinking, because surely mountains don't blink.

From here, we begin to move. Inhale arms reach up, exhale fold forward, bend your knees, place your fingertips to the floor, inhale look up, exhale step your left leg back, knee down, inhale arms reach . . . it goes on like this for a while. I feel awkward at first, but after a while, my body settles in and moves more easily, as though it instinctively knows what to do next. I am naturally strong and flexible, which makes me feel like maybe I'm not so out of place after all.

Then the teacher comes over and tells me to remove my socks. I look at him for a long moment, feeling embarrassed, before I reluctantly do what I am told. I watch as his gaze alights on the bandages covering my toes and heels. He raises an eyebrow again and then simply says, "Push down into the floor . . . and spread your toes!" I do, grateful he didn't say anything more, and I marvel that such a simple instruction could make me feel more connected to the ground beneath me.

The teacher leads us from pose to pose, and except for the constant nausea, a slight headache, and an overall achiness in my muscles, I feel pretty good. Finally, he tells us to "prepare for Savasana." I look around as everyone begins to hit the floor, close their eyes, and settle in. I join them, and completely pass out. The clanging of those chimes startles me awake. I sit up cross-legged, like the others, and bring my palms into prayer. Another chant is followed by an OM—my first OM. The teacher ends class with a "namaste," which the students repeat back, some with heads bowed, others with their whole body folded forward toward the floor. I just sit there, staring at the deities on the altar in the front of the room, feeling both settled and utterly sick to my stomach. I roll up my mat, nod a thank you to the teacher, and leave. In the bathroom downstairs, I lean over the toilet and puke.

▼

I continued going to Integral, mostly because I liked telling the people at Life Café that I did yoga too. I enjoyed the movements though. The nausea I felt initially was apparently a sign that my system was cleansing itself from my diet, my smoking habit, and other environmental factors I was subjected to every day, like the exhaust from cars. The teacher said that it was normal for me to feel sick before feeling better because the increased blood flow was drawing toxins out of my organs and back through my bloodstream. Sounded about right to me.

Practicing asana made me feel strong, fit, and capable. I liked that I could so easily accomplish poses that seemed to challenge the other students in the room. I really enjoyed finding the people in the room who seemed most "advanced" and rolling out my mat next to theirs. It motivated me to work hard and move my body into more and more complicated shapes. Doing asana was fun! My confidence was building. Conversely, I merely tolerated the chanting, was deeply bored by the meditation, and, more often than not, zoned out completely during the prayers.

And yoga wasn't giving me the transcendent experiences that David and Sharon had talked about. I wasn't experiencing the "God within" or "altered states of awareness beyond any drug you've ever taken," or anything even remotely like that. Maybe I wasn't doing it right? Sometimes there'd be discussions at the beginning of the class, called dharma talks, about Spirit. I'd sit tall like a good yogi and listen, nodding my head here and there in agreement, but these talks didn't really do it for me either. I tried to hide my restlessness. I just wanted to move my body.

Although I didn't notice many changes in my personality, and wasn't exactly having glimpses into enlightened states, the more I practiced, the more aware I became about how my behaviors impacted my physical health. Eventually, I didn't want to put things into my mouth (or up my nose) that didn't feel good—and that included alcohol, junk food, and drugs. Smoking was the last really bad habit to go. I loved a good cigarette. First thing in the morning, I'd reach over to my nightstand, fumble a cigarette out of the pack of Marlboro Reds, light it, and enjoy the first inhale of nicotine as it passed down into my lungs. I'd swing my legs over the side of the bed; my hair a knotted, frizzy mess; and watch myself in the mirror French-inhaling the smoke from my partly opened lips up into my nose. That was the sexiest move I had. I especially loved a good smoke immediately after yoga class. I would literally have a butt hanging from my mouth, lighter at the ready, as I was leaving the studio. That thing would be lit the second the door closed behind me.

Then one day, about a year later, I was sitting on a curb in Jersey, waiting for the 197 Express to take me back to the city. I put a Marlboro to my lips and inhaled. Instead of drawing the smoke into my lungs, I immediately coughed and sputtered, and exhaled it out as fast as I could. The taste in my mouth was foul. I coughed some more, my lungs tight and my throat sore. I smelled the pack thinking maybe they were stale. They smelled exactly as they always did. Without even glancing at my cigarette to mark the ceremony of the moment, I flicked the butt into the street. I knew that was that. I tossed the rest of the pack into the garbage and never smoked again.

▼

After a long night of tending bar at Shescape, a lesbian party that floated to different clubs around the city, I managed to open my eyes around noon. I lay there staring at the ceiling, my boyfriend asleep nearby. Although his body was warm and inviting, I moved farther away, curled on to my side, and stared out the window, watching as Manhattan got on with her day. I heard the cars and people below heading toward their destination. *At least they're going somewhere,* I thought. I sighed, pulled the sheets off me and sat on the edge of the bed, my head in my hands, the smell of smoke and beer still in my hair. I was twenty-two years old, living with yet another boyfriend, and stuck. I didn't feel particularly connected to anything. I painted, took acting classes, and attended random college courses in philosophy and writing at The New School. I participated in a few social movements, attending rallies and protests for causes I believed in. I was a part of a theater company and even did performing arts in the parks and on the streets in the Lower East Side. I worked in some of the hippest nightclubs in the world and had plenty of friends. But I didn't know what I was going to do with my life or what I was truly passionate about. I felt purposeless. *What if I never make a living doing anything other than waiting tables or tending bar?* It was hard work, the hours sucked, and I was really bad at it. I knew half the reason I got these jobs was because I was cute in a 1980s punk sort of way, not because I was any good at service. I felt lucky to have these jobs and make as much money as I did, but I didn't want to be in the service industry, and I was afraid that I didn't have any other choice because I had no other skills, no education. Without either, what could someone like me do? I looked over at my boyfriend. *He made a decent living. Maybe I should just marry him . . . ?*

As I sat there, I could feel my anxiety rise, a sensation of restlessness moving just below the layers of my skin. It was such a familiar feeling, something I had known since I was a kid. I got up and quietly paced around the apartment, randomly straightening things up. I went into another room and turned on the TV; the sound in the room made me feel less alone. I knew that if I called any number of friends, I could hang with them. Maybe we could grab an afternoon drink or smoke a joint? It had been a while since I partied, so it might be fun to let loose a little. I imagined the scene, pictured myself throwing back a shot of tequila, the warmth of the liquor pouring down my throat, the heady, light feeling I'd experience as it made its way into my bloodstream. The idea felt good for a moment; in fact, just thinking about it made my heartbeat slow down. I stood there considering it, then shook it off. I thought about how I'd feel later. Not good. I really didn't want to drink or do drugs anymore. I thought maybe I could hook up with that guy I had recently stopped seeing. He had a girlfriend, but we'd often meet up on the roof of his apartment building downtown and screw while looking out over the city. It was okay that we were hooking up since I had a boyfriend too, so it didn't really feel like cheating. I picked up the phone to dial his number, sat there for a moment, holding the receiver to my ear, and then put it back into its cradle. I didn't want to lie anymore, and I also didn't want to have sex with someone I didn't care about or who really didn't care about me. Crap. I considered getting something to eat. Sometimes that made me feel better. I could go to the Odessa diner on Avenue A and have a massive plate of cheese pierogi pan-fried in butter with sour cream and applesauce, like my grandmother made. Whenever I felt sad, she'd cook up a vat, and I always felt good afterward. Maybe that's what I needed.

I sat down on the floor in the middle of my apartment, frozen with indecision. I knew any one of those choices would make me feel better in the short run, but I suddenly knew that whichever one I chose would make me feel worse later. I picked at the skin on my big toe, peeling it back in thin shards until it started to bleed.

Not knowing what else to do, I looked around, picked up yesterday's sweats and T-shirt off the floor, threw them on, and headed out the door, trudging my way through the snow on the cold, gray, miserable day to Integral Yoga. I walked in, said hi to the receptionist, kicked off my boots, went upstairs, and rolled out my mat. I managed to slog through my practice, somehow, but I felt distracted. All I could do was methodically move from one pose to another.

The teacher wasn't having it.

▼

"Feel your feet on the floor, thighs lift, tailbone in, breathe!" the teacher commands. I am limp in my poses, and he keeps adjusting me and fine-tuning my shapes. The changes he's asking me to make are uncomfortable, requiring more strength than I have, and I can hardly keep my balance. He keeps saying, "Seane, focus, ground, breathe! You're not breathing!" I think, *Obviously I'm breathing, asshole, otherwise I'd be dead. He is picking on me!* Every time I go into a pose, he adjusts it, making it harder for me to hold. My body feels thick and tight. I feel nauseous, and my thoughts are all over the place. I think about drugs, drinking, my boyfriend, my lover, my aching body, my life, and what a weak, lazy pig I am that I can't hold the poses. *I even suck at that now*, I think. *Great. What else?*

"Breathe!" he continues. The breathing in the room is rhythmic and deep; mine is shallow and impatient. I glance at the male student nearby and wonder if he thinks I'm pretty. During the floor work, I wonder what it would be like to have sex with him, and by the time we go up into Shoulderstand, we're married with children.

During Savasana, I fall asleep, as usual, but this time, my snoring wakes me up. I feel disoriented and embarrassed, hoping my new husband hasn't heard me. I place my hands into namaste when instructed to, bow my head, chant a feeble OM with the class, roll up my mat, and split.

Outside it has started to snow. New York looks eerily beautiful when it snows; the white flakes cover the dirt and grime, and everything looks crisp, clean, and enchanted. It's cold, so I pull my coat tighter around my body, inhaling the fresh air, allowing the snowflakes to rest on my eyelashes. The air feels chilly in my lungs. I exhale it out completely, watching as the white mist rises from my mouth, and then take another full breath in. Suddenly, I stop in my tracks, exhale, and wait. I look around, taking everything in as if it were all new to me. Which it isn't, of course. I've walked this particular street countless times. I can't seem to describe what I feel; I just know something's off. I pat my pockets for my keys. Check. I open my bag to see if I have my wallet. Yep. Everything's where it should be. I stand in that spot for a long time, trying to get a sense of what's going on. I look up at the large clock above Greenwich Avenue just as the sun is setting, and I see its pale pink reflection against the white backdrop.

Slowly, I smile. Something *is* different. That something is me.

I stand there, my arms to my sides, my face still turned up toward the pinkish sky, and I know that everything in my life is truly okay. That everything is unfolding perfectly, and I am exactly where I'm supposed to be. The word "trust" keeps bubbling up from deep inside. I speak the word, quietly. "Trust," I whisper again, squinting now toward Jersey, to where I was raised. "Trust."

My heart is full, so absolute and satisfied. I wonder: *Could it have been the yoga practice that made me feel so content, open, and unafraid? How is that possible? How could asana change my fear? How could practicing a bunch of poses make me feel, I don't know, like happy? Actually, exactly like happy.*

Most days I leave yoga feeling pretty good, but this time is different. This is beyond the body. Nothing has changed, I still have no sense of purpose, but somehow I know it will all work out. I place my hands on my heart, the snow settling on my face, and smile. I am immensely grateful.

The next day when I wake up, the anxiety's back. Not as much as the day before, but still, negative thoughts begin to spin in my head. I automatically consider my go-to options to change the discomfort—drinking, eating, or getting laid. I sit there, staring at the floor, imagining all my options. Finally I take a breath, get dressed, and go to yoga.

TEACHINGS FROM 13TH STREET
ASANA, KOSHAS, AND NIYAMAS

Yoga has a way of giving you what you want at first . . . and then later presenting what you need, whether you're ready to accept it or not. Sometimes these changes are obvious and smack you right in the face. Other times, the shifts are subtle, sneaking up on you and catching you completely off guard. That's what happened to me that day after yoga class when I experienced pure, unadulterated happiness and ease.

Yoga had cut through my resistance and offered me the steadiness and peace that comes from simply being. For a few fleeting moments, I got a glimpse of the power of yoga to move us from attachment to freedom, from illusion to understanding. And I felt something I couldn't define at first. I felt whole. Yoga was showing me what was possible if I committed to doing the work, if I accepted its invitation into my own awakening.

Of course the feeling didn't last, but I did get a respite from the anxiety, fear, and insecurity that I'd experienced off and on for most of my life. Looking back, I can see that the moment of awareness I encountered on the streets of New York City was an invitation to begin the journey toward self-discovery, to bear witness to all parts of me, and to tend to my own humanity—the light parts as well as the shadow parts I didn't want to acknowledge. This journey is the evolution of the soul. But at that moment? I just felt happy and content.

Without knowing the how, what, or why of any of yoga's inner workings, I had experienced the integration of my whole being—every layer of it. Yoga calls these layers *koshas*, or sheaths, a reminder that we are more than just the physical body we can see and touch. We are body, breath, mind, intuition, and radiant awareness. So what does all that mean on a practical level? How do all those things contribute to our evolution? To our awakening? I hadn't a clue then. All I knew was I went to yoga, sat still, breathed on cue, moved around a bit, sat still again, and laid down. Underneath all of this, apparently, my relationship to my body, mind, and heart was undergoing quite a transformation.

THE KOSHAS

Even when we're not aware of it, doing yoga profoundly affects all parts of our being—our body, breath, mind, heart, and soul, better known in yoga as the koshas. As a body-based meditation, yoga invites us to focus, stabilize, and move with more awareness. Nothing within us stands alone—we are living, breathing, thinking, feeling beings imbued with Universal Consciousness or Divine Essence.

Annamaya Kosha (The Physical or Food Body)

My journey toward spiritual evolution began with the physical body, which is most often where it all begins. Why? Because we start with what we know: what we can hear, feel, taste, touch, and smell. It's tangible. The Yoga Sutras say we need to take care of our "container"—our bones, muscles, joints, and tissues. We must cleanse it, strengthen it, and bring more flexibility to the spine through asana practice so we can sit in meditation or prayer for longer periods of time without distraction or discomfort.

Many people begin yoga with less-than-healthy diets and habits, and find the body isn't willing to put up with all that for very long. Feeling nauseous is often their first clue that they need to detoxify and rethink their choices. That certainly happened to me. Because of my diet and all the drugs, drinking, and smoking I had been doing, my cells, tissues, and organs carried impurities that I needed to bathe and cleanse through asana and pranayama. And then, of course, I needed to actually change my diet and my lifestyle choices in order to maintain good health. The physical cleansing of the body is a vital step on the spiritual path toward wholeness, because, as B.K.S. Iyengar, the leading authority in contemporary yoga, used to say, "You can't build a temple on quicksand."

Focusing on the body can keep you in the present moment, grounded in your experience, able to investigate what's going on physically. My yoga teacher was right to insist that I feel my feet on the earth. He could see the tension in my body, my discomfort, and almost demanded that I move the energy down and allow the earth to support me. Being in the *annamaya kosha* can show you where your tension is held and give you a glimpse of what may lie buried under that tension—the traumas and the suffering you may have been harboring for many lifetimes.

Of course, focusing on the body is quite different from becoming attached to what it can do. And attached I was—deeply. At first, the physical practice gave me an appreciation for my body that I hadn't had before. I was surprised by its strength and its agility. But it didn't take long before my ability on the mat gave me the external approval I craved, an identity I could be proud of. It served and stroked my ego. When we let the mind dictate what our practice should look like or say about us, we've moved from a body-based practice to an ego-based one.

Pranamaya Kosha (The Energy Body)

Of course I couldn't have had the physical practice I was so attached to without learning how to breathe correctly. I didn't know much about what went on under the surface, but I did know that the more I practiced the deep breathing exercises (pranayama) in yoga class, the better I felt.

Your breath, your life-force, is the current that runs through this subtle energy pathway; it's known as *prana*, or *chi* in Chinese medicine. Most people think of it as the breath, but it's really more than that. It's the delivery system that brings vital energy to every cell, channel, muscle, nook, and cranny in the body. It makes sure that all of your biological processes, which include breathing, circulation, and digestion, function properly. When prana gets deregulated—whether blocked, stagnant, or overstimulated—it can mess you up pretty thoroughly.

My Integral Yoga teacher knew what he was doing when he scolded me for not breathing. You cannot find freedom in the body, he said, you cannot feel at ease in your skin, without paying attention to the breath. At the same time, doing asana in a way that opens up the spaces in your body gives the breath more freedom to distribute prana. They are clearly linked.

He would often point out that thoughts and emotions move through the body on the wave of prana, so it's not unusual to notice that our emotions affect the rhythm and quality of our breath. I noticed, for example, that when I was angry, scared, or even distracted, my breath became agitated or shortened, and I couldn't hold poses the same way. I couldn't balance or even flow through a yoga sequence very smoothly.

I discovered that changing my habits and my diet, including getting more fresh air and being out in the sunshine—which is the ultimate source of prana—doing acupuncture, and eating plenty of raw fruits and veggies, made me feel better and more aligned. My energy increased, which impacted my mood and my ability to be more open and receptive.

Manomaya Kosha (The Mental Body)

According to the yogic tradition, the central nervous system, which comprises our brain and spinal cord, processes and sends information from the *manomaya kosha* (the mental body) to the annamaya kosha (the physical body). In other words, the body and mind are connected through the agency of the breath. The manomaya kosha is the active, reactive, and not-so-discerning mind that flits from thing to thing and, if you're lucky, quiets down through asana, pranayama, and meditation practices. It is deeply influenced by what you see or experience—and can make split decisions based on that—but it's not so good at processing any of it.

I was quite familiar with the manomaya kosha; in fact, that's where I often got stuck. Because of my anxiety and my impulse to lessen it through the use of substances and unhealthy behavior, I found it difficult to put my thoughts to rest. The antidote to "monkey mind"—the Buddhist term for a restless mind—is concentration, which isn't really designed to shut down the mind. Rather, it can bring you clarity and insight, and cultivate (maybe even widen) the gap between your thoughts, which brings more ease. Any form of concentration or meditation can be very difficult if your mind never shuts up—like mine—and you don't know how to slow it down. Asana can help you move any agitation out of your mind and into your body so you can identify it, notice where it lives, and release it.

Vijnanamaya Kosha
(The Wisdom Body)

The *vijnanamaya kosha* is your inner wisdom. Awakening this kosha means getting in touch with your discerning, or intuitive, mind. That allows you to direct your life from your heart instead of your head, which means you can make more ethical, moral, and mindful choices, free from the impulse of any addictions, compulsions, and desires. It provides the pause between your thoughts and your actions that you need in order to show up for yourself and others with more patience and generosity and less judgment. It can help you see where you limit yourself by your actions, fears, or unprocessed traumas.

I rarely experienced this kosha on a conscious level at the beginning. I was highly intuitive, but I hadn't really developed or nurtured this skill. Wisdom and intuition require trust and self confidence. And I didn't have much of either. I was too busy struggling with the impulses that led me to make unhealthy decisions. My ego was stronger than my will to change, and I couldn't see how my judgments were impaired. My desire to smoke, drink, do drugs, eat mindlessly, and act out sexually gave me a way to numb out, a surefire method to separate myself from my discomfort. How could I trust my intuition when the beliefs I had about myself kept me from the truth of who I was?

Meditation and quiet reflection help engage the wisdom, or discerning, mind. The yamas and niyamas, the first of the eight limbs, are designed to help us access the vijnanamaya kosha. Learning to breathe in and out of our heart, reading spiritual texts—the "food" that nourishes the intellect and fosters a deeper understanding of ourselves and others—and practicing kindness and non-judgment all help develop our intuition. Through these practices, we can begin to experience the whole of life—even the painful or grief-filled moments—with more compassion and even objectivity. It is through the vijnanamaya kosha that we develop clarity of the mind, greater intuitive understanding, and increased willpower.

Anandamaya Kosha
(The Bliss Body)

The subtlest of the energy bodies, the *anandamaya kosha*, connects our ordinary awareness with our highest Self or Spirit. Although it exists in all of us, most of us aren't aware of this layer of our being. The anandamaya kosha represents all-knowing wisdom, radiant awareness, transcendent illumination—in other words, pure bliss. You experience the bliss body when you suddenly and inexplicably feel at ease, when you connect with someone so deeply you can't tell where you leave off and the other person begins. You experience it when you enter into a yoga pose and after moving around, tweaking the alignment, and getting settled in, you simply receive the pose. You're no longer *doing* the pose; you *are* the pose.

All five of the koshas are activated whenever you do asana, even the bliss body. Yoga invites you to experience the anandamaya kosha through devotion to God, through selfless service out in the world, and by accessing the God within.

Looking back on what happened that day after class, I realize that I truly experienced all five sheaths at once, in a simple but quite profound way. As I gazed up at the pale pink reflection of the setting sun through that large clock face on Greenwich Avenue, everything came together; everything was perfect. My heart felt full, my body and mind calm and clear, my breath barely discernible. There was no separation between the experience and the "me" doing the experiencing. I was, for that moment, connected to everything around me. I felt grateful. And for once in my life, I didn't argue with my experience; I didn't minimize it by reminding myself that I still had no purpose, that I was still basically an anxious mess. I simply received what was happening, fully present to the moment I was in, and felt at peace.

NIYAMAS

In those precious moments when our doubts and agitations drop away, we can sometimes glimpse what is possible—and what is already true. If we truly pay attention, yoga can show us how to take better care of ourselves, and perhaps even teach us how to love ourselves more. The way it does that is through the niyamas, the second of the eight limbs of yoga. These five "observances" encourage us to engage with ourselves as consciously as we can, so we can notice the places in our lives where we're out of sync with our true nature and commit over and over again to this self-inquiry, with patience and generosity. As I said earlier, these mindfulness practices help strengthen our connection to ourselves and ask us to reflect on who we are and the attachments we have to our own stories. And, of course, yoga asks us to approach each one of these observances lovingly (ahimsa).

Saucha (Purification)

First on the niyama list, *saucha* means to purify or cleanse, to rid the body and the mind of anything that causes suffering. This niyama goes hand-in-hand with the first yama, ahimsa. On a physical level, it means keeping your surroundings clean and organized, something that my young self pretty much failed to do. It also means treating your body with respect, shying away from foods (and other substances) that don't agree with your constitution and focusing on fresh, organic, local foods, if possible. I was getting better at that.

Saucha also encourages you to get clear on what thoughts and emotions you allow to enter your mind. A cluttered mind is neither clear nor calm. Saucha asks the questions: As thoughts and feelings come up, which ones do you hold on to, which ones

do you feed until they grow much bigger than they were ever intended to be? And which ones keep you stuck and unable to move forward? Think of saucha as "decluttering" the mind, ridding it of any judgments, fears, excuses, and unhealthy habits so you can shine the light on your inner radiance and the God within yourself and others.

I got a rather jarring saucha experience the very first day I stepped onto my mat. Almost the minute I started moving and breathing, I felt nauseous, and it only got worse during the practice; right after class, I threw up. Yoga asana and the conscious breathing we were doing made me critically aware of my choices and behaviors, especially the ones that were self-sabotaging. Although I occasionally entertained the idea of returning to my old standbys as methods of self-soothing, the truth was they no longer appealed. The yogis were right: impurities in our physical environment, including drugs, alcohol, poor diet, and environmental stressors, do affect our mental and emotional states. As I practiced asana and pranayama, both of which increase circulation and help the body process and eliminate these impurities, I no longer wanted to keep adding more stuff that would need to be cleansed.

Santosha (Contentment)

Ah, contentment. Being satisfied with what is. Some even translate *santosha* as "happiness or delight" and connect it to the yamas satya and asteya (truthfulness and non-stealing). Think of santosha as present-moment acceptance, welcoming all of your experiences and relationships and seeing them as integral to who you are. It is understanding your narrative but not being limited by what you tell yourself.

I got a glimpse into santosha when I experienced that deep contentment, or happiness, on that cold, snowy day in front of the clock. In that one moment, I experienced the deep peace that comes from being completely present, not needing anything to be different. I knew then that I would be just fine; in fact, I could see that everything was perfect just the way it was, including me.

Contentment arrives when our wholeness comes from within. If we define ourselves by how much money we make, how many friends we have, or how many things we own, we can never be satisfied. There's never enough out there to fill the emptiness inside because what we're actually lacking is a sense of our own goodness, a sense that yes, we *are* enough. Experiencing santosha means letting go of the past. It means refraining from condemning yourself for not being cooler, smarter, richer, sexier, or even nicer. It means freeing the mind of all the "if onlys," "shouldas," and "wouldas" that cloud your thinking. Once that happens, once you experience a taste of happiness or delight, you may find that you're more patient with yourself and that you can acknowledge your gifts and accept your limitations as challenges.

Tapas (Discipline)

There are so many translations of *tapas*—"heat," "discipline," "simplicity," "willpower." Following saucha and santosha, tapas as simplicity and discipline continues to invite you to do a little internal housekeeping, to shed all your excuses, all your emotional baggage and excesses, and to just show up for your practice and for your life. Tapas as heat gives you the focus and the willpower you need to keep practicing consistently, to face and work through your difficulties, and to emerge, hopefully, with more self-awareness and self-love. And, finally, tapas as practice reminds you that this is indeed a *practice*, that you need only focus on one or two things at a time so as not to get overwhelmed and give up. Those small steps can strengthen your body and increase your confidence.

I definitely practiced tapas because it often took incredible discipline not to fall into old mindless habits when I got discouraged or felt anxious. It sometimes took fierce determination and razor-like focus to disentangle myself from the pull of my old go-to behaviors and drag my ass to yoga, even when I knew it would ground me, even when I knew it would release the accumulated energy blocking entrance into the deeper realms of my being. It eventually allowed me to cultivate the conscious awareness to stop indulging in unhealthy habits and impulses. By committing to practice, I eventually found a simpler, gentler way to ease my anxiety and make me feel better.

Svadhyaya (Self-Study)

The literal translation of *svadhyaya* is "self-study," which invites us to examine our own nature, to get to know the Divine presence at the core of our being.

It is self-awareness *without judgment*. To start, we must become conscious of all the self-sabotaging actions and thoughts that serve as roadblocks on the path and then guide the mind toward more healthful ones. How do we do that when we haven't a clue what propels us to act or think in certain ways—some skillful and others not so much?

The first step is to remember that this kind of self-awareness requires no makeovers or do-overs; instead, it pulls back the veil of doubt, anxiety, insecurity, fear, blame, and shame, and reveals our true nature—which is basic goodness and, of course, love. You can start by turning to the wisdom found in sacred or spiritual texts, which can give you insights into human nature and inspire you to be more mindful. Then you can move inward, with compassion, getting to know and understand yourself a little bit more. You can do that on and off your mat. Without svadhyaya, it's easy to get caught up in the ego's delight at "performing" poses, and yoga becomes nothing more than a physical distraction. Svadhyaya, on the other hand, wants you to notice when your actions and thoughts are out of harmony with your purest intentions, to notice when you're doing things that could set you apart from others. When your mind wanders and your actions are less than skillful, such self-awareness allows you to gently come back into integrity, come back to your essence. Above all, svadhyaya cultivates the wisdom mind and encourages you to dwell in the bliss body where you can feel the presence of your Divine Spirit.

Using mantra meditation—many yoga experts encourage silently reciting the Sanskrit phrase *so hum*, which means "that, I am"—is one of the best ways to practice svadhyaya. Inhaling *so* and exhaling *hum* will fill the mind with sound so it's less distracted by mindless chatter and able to experience true Self-awareness (or Divine Consciousness).

When I first started going to Integral Yoga, I hadn't started looking inward enough to understand that there might be guidance available to me. I did get inklings from time to time that suggested my actions were either healthful or harmful. But I was still pretty shut down emotionally and definitely suspicious of spiritual practice. You certainly wouldn't catch me reading the Bible or any other sacred text—I could barely sit still during meditation, and I zoned out

when someone led a yoga class in anything that resembled a prayer. But during my "happy" experience, I felt something beyond the physical, beyond my ability to explain it away. And, I felt oddly confident that, if I kept at it, all this yoga, meditation, and breathwork could help me understand the complexities of the human experience and be willing to explore the depths of my own interior—with a lot less resistance.

Ishvara Pranidhana (Devotion or Surrender)

To dedicate yourself—and surrender—to what yoga calls the all-pervading Consciousness (or Divine Essence) is the ideal of *ishvara pranidhana*. Surrender doesn't mean giving up or feeling defeated. It means giving yourself over to a higher purpose, seeing the "bigger picture," getting out of the way in order for the soul to evolve. It requires that you surrender to the mystery and trust that the Universe will present what you need, when you need it.

Ishvara pranidhana, on the mat, means to practice without being attached to the outcome, to focus on the process and not be concerned with the results.

You may not be able to control what's going on in your life, but you can control how you think and feel about it all. But ishvara pranidhana means even more than all that. It means that you must dedicate the merits of your actions, of your practice, to something bigger than yourself. Everything you do must in some small way benefit all life.

There was no part of my reality that accepted or even understood this one. It was all I could do, literally and figuratively, to stand on my own two feet, breathe properly, and take my place on the mat. That was plenty! But when I stood there on Greenwich Avenue, wrapped in happiness, I got a taste of what's possible. Sure, I would continue to have moments of deep insecurity and anxiety. We all do—this is not a one-and-done. But on that corner, I felt *something*, and that *something* helped me understand a bit of what Billy had been talking about. I accepted things as they were—at that very moment—without trying to justify, explain, or change anything. I was happy, and I was at peace.

BREATHE AND EVERYTHING CHANGES

EVEN THOUGH I STILL enjoyed periods of contentment as my yoga practice deepened, I would get flashes of awareness in the quiet moments of meditation that were uncomfortable and disturbing. Thoughts of my childhood would suddenly arise seemingly out of nowhere. Sometimes my mental meanderings took the form of an inner dialogue; other times, images emerged, feelings lingered. I'd try to shake off the thoughts, but they kept coming. I didn't *want* to think about stuff that made me uncomfortable. And I certainly didn't want to feel any of it.

Before, when this happened, I could change the script easily, numbing out my pain and frustration with inappropriate behaviors and a menu of drugs and alcohol. But now those choices didn't have the same soothing effect they once had. Quite the opposite actually. Was yoga suddenly messing with me? Why was all the breathing, moving, and sitting stirring old shit up? Shit that I hadn't thought about for years. Of course I had no clue then that yoga would place what needed to be acknowledged front and center until the body, mind, and heart could receive it, assimilate it, and then let it go. All I knew was that "stuff was coming up," as the teacher sometimes warned us could happen. But I didn't like it, and I needed to do something about it.

I decided to try therapy.

Therapy wasn't something I was raised to believe in. I definitely came from a no-nonsense, "get over yourself" kind of environment. Therapy meant something was wrong with you or that you were a spoiled narcissist who could afford to whine to a stranger about your "problems." But in my mind, there *wasn't* anything wrong with me. Sure, I had problems like everyone else, but nothing I couldn't manage. And I was certainly not spoiled. I didn't have that kind of upbringing.

But the fact was, I had suffered from a persistent, low-grade anxiety ever since I was a kid. I just had good coping skills, and I could easily mask my feelings with humor and charm. Inwardly, I often felt shaky and edgy. I twirled my hair, picked at my cuticles, and peeled the bottoms of my feet, my anxiety craving some form of expression. Finally, my friend Kevin, a big believer in personal transformation, convinced me to see his therapist, a man named Norman. Norman was a Gestalt therapist and a Zen Buddhist; he was also the first person to introduce me to the phrase obsessive-compulsive disorder (OCD).

I never knew that the repetitive behaviors and rituals I had done since I was a little girl had a name. They actually didn't back then, but by the time I began seeing Norman, psychologists used the acronym OCD to describe a variety of obsessive behaviors, some of which I exhibited. I thought I was just quirky and that these compulsive rituals were unique to me.

Ever since I was about seven years old, I loved the balance and synergy of even numbers, especially fours and eights. Whenever I touched objects an even number of times, I immediately felt more relaxed and grounded. When I didn't, and if the numbers were odd, I became ill at ease in my body and obsessive in my thoughts. Over time, I developed superstitions around my repetitive-counting compulsion, which caused my pattern-making behaviors to escalate. I often worried. A lot. I thought about death. Often. Especially my parents' death. I was certain that something horrible would happen to me, or someone I loved, if I neglected to perform my rituals. Those rituals, in fact, became a matter of great importance and urgency, the one way I could ensure that those I loved remained safe.

I counted my blinking, my swallowing, the number of times I or someone else said "good-bye," "I love you," or any other sentiment. God forbid they only said it three times! I would badger them or say, "What did you just say?" until they added the fourth proclamation. Of course, I could never step on a crack in the sidewalk, and games like hopscotch secretly terrified me because I couldn't chance landing on one of the lines. If I did, I would immediately and subtly begin "patterning" so I could prevent getting "jinxed" and stave off some imaginary doom.

By the time I reached puberty, my obsessions had gotten worse and more complex. Lord help me if someone accidentally brushed up against one side of my body or knocked into me. I would instantly feel the panic set in and wonder how I could get them to brush against or knock into my other side without it being weird. It was always weird. I would awkwardly bump up against people, say I'm sorry, but actually feel relieved if I managed to replicate the action that had happened on the other side. My brothers would mess with me. As soon as they noticed I was getting distracted or was watching TV, they'd start poking me on one shoulder and then whisper in my ear, "You out of balance yet?" My whole body would tense, and I'd beg them to poke the other shoulder to "balance me out." When they'd refuse, anxiety and dread would flood my body, and I'd go crying to my mother until she made them do it. It was also during this time that I started cutting my feet.

I always thought I'd eventually grow out of my odd habits. Instead, when I moved to New York City, the stress of being in an intense environment away from my family, especially my mother—the only person I felt truly safe with—meant that my symptoms worsened.

I lived on the fourth floor of a walk-up on Avenue B. Every day when I left my apartment, I'd have to count the fifty-six stairs between my front door and the bottom landing. As soon I got to the bottom, I'd turn around, go back upstairs, and check to see if I'd locked the door. It didn't matter if I knew the door was locked—of course it was locked!—I had to do it anyway. I would count the fifty-six steps on the way back up, check the door, and then count the fifty-six steps back down. I had to repeat this ritual four times. Every day. No matter what.

Soon I noticed a need to pattern on the mat too. When the teacher would tell us to press all four points of the foot down, I had to feel that action fully and evenly before I could move on. Alignment in the poses made me acutely aware that my body wasn't exactly the same on both sides. One of my hips was higher than the other. My spine had a slight curvature to it, making my right shoulder drop lower than the left. The imbalance caused pangs of anxiety to rise right in the middle of Mountain Pose, when all I was doing was standing with my feet together! My compulsive behaviors were only getting worse, and my anxiety associated with them was becoming more of a distraction, especially since I had quit partying and self-medicating.

I certainly hoped that Norman could help me get to the bottom of all this.

▼

One day in therapy, Norman begins talking about trauma and the unique way the nervous system responds to what he calls "deregulation." And then he says, "I believe you do these rituals to stave off the discomfort you feel in your body as a result of your trauma. It's your way of self-regulating."

"What trauma? I've never experienced trauma."

Norman just stares at me blankly, waiting for me to figure it out. I quietly stare back.

"Your molestation?" he says finally.

"My molestation? That was no big deal at all. I rarely think about it. And, anyway, what does that have to do with me counting things?"

Norman falls silent again. Waiting.

When I was six years old, I was sexually molested by a distant adult relative. He was young and cool and someone whom I adored and trusted.

When it happened, I experienced what anyone who was being violated in that way might, especially a child: fear, of course; shame, without a doubt; but there was another sensation that confused me greatly. Pleasure. What was happening was horrible; even at six I knew it was wrong. I didn't know what it was, exactly, but I did know I wanted it to stop. At the same time, though, my body was flooded with sensations that felt oddly pleasurable, and I had no way of assigning meaning to them.

But back then, I did what so many others do in such a situation: I dissociated. I checked out and separated myself from my body. I didn't do this consciously. It just happened. I observed what was going on as though it were happening to someone else. I was there, but gone. I couldn't move. I couldn't speak. I couldn't feel. I just floated above myself, watching without alarm or empathy.

But truthfully, I hadn't really thought much about what had happened for a really long time—and I certainly never considered it traumatic. I had only mentioned my experience to Norman once, in passing. I didn't cry or get angry. Sitting in front of him now, I reiterate that my life hasn't really been affected by it.

Norman doesn't agree.

"Your molestation is trauma," he says. "Trauma is any event you experience that leaves you feeling helpless, out of control, in despair, unable to defend yourself, or powerless to respond. Each of us reacts to trauma in different ways depending on the severity of the event and our ability to process what happened."

I just stare at him.

The thing is, I don't feel helpless, in despair, or out of control. I don't really feel anything. But I am willing to dive in and see what I can learn. The longer I work with Norman, the more I begin to see how being molested really has impacted my psyche and my body. I learn that since I didn't know how to process, or even understand, the fear, shame, guilt, rage, and confusion I felt, I simply shoved all those emotions down, where they have remained trapped in my body ever since and have formed a deep layer of protective tension. Tension that I have long relied on to actually help me feel safe, or at least alert. Tension that practicing yoga had begun to release.

My OCD had started shortly after I was molested, so had the anxiety. My patterning, Norman says, has always been a way to find balance in the chaos. That's news to me. I just know that it helps decrease the unease I feel and makes me calmer and more grounded. Anxiety makes my heart beat too fast, my skin tingle, and my muscles ache. It brings warmth to my face and chest and a stabby feeling in my stomach. But when I touch things in even numbers, those symptoms subside, and I feel in control again. As a young person, patterning was my drug of choice—at least until I chose to do actual drugs. No matter what I did to alter the deep discomfort I felt, however, I was never conscious of what was at its core or how deeply repressed the emotions were that lived within me.

My molestation at six years old had not been the last time I was assaulted. Men regularly exposed themselves in front of me or touched me. It happened in the New York Public Library, on subways, in parking lots. Every time it happened, I would feel afraid, get dizzy, freeze up, and then numb out—classic dissociation. What I couldn't do was take action, which was beyond frustrating to me.

So I would move through the world, as most women do, anticipating the inevitable assault—including rape—that was certain to come when my "luck" finally ran out. I was sure that when it did, I would not be able to fight or flee. Because my dissociation had kept me in some sort of emotional disconnect, I would probably freeze or fold and allow whatever my assaulter wanted to happen to happen—just like I'd done when I was six.

I work hard with Norman, trying to reconcile the events of my childhood and understand the impact that sexual molestation and harassment has had on my psyche and my life. It takes time, but I eventually become open to healing my trauma. I can finally see how it is connected to my obsessive attachments and patterning, and I want more than anything to understand and heal it.

Norman ascribes to the theory of "detachment." He tells me that whenever a big feeling comes up, I should witness it, be present to it, and then let it go. So I spend a lot of time "detaching" from my rage and shame, which feels good and even helpful at times. Of course it does. Detachment for me is simply a code word for dissociation, and Norman has inadvertently given me another method I can use to bypass uncomfortable feelings. Obviously, that's not what he intended, but that's how I interpret it. I can describe how I feel, I can discuss what I feel, but by practicing "detachment," I don't actually have to feel it.

Although Norman helps me understand my OCD, the path to healing it begins, not surprisingly, in a yoga class.

I'm in Downward-Facing Dog, and the teacher accidentally kicks my right heel as he walks past me. My body immediately feels out of balance—the sensation in my right heel is almost unbearable—and I begin to inwardly panic. I somehow keep moving through the poses, but the whole time I'm obsessing over how I can get him to kick my left heel. I think maybe when I say goodbye, I could "accidentally" trip near him and hit his foot with my left heel. But then I would have to hit his right foot twice—with both of mine—to even things out. *But, what if . . . and then what . . . and . . . ?* My mind is spinning, and the oh-so-familiar anxiety builds. Meanwhile, no one around me has a clue that anything is amiss. As far as they're concerned, I'm just doing my practice.

Then, seemingly at random, the teacher says to the whole class, "Breathe and everything changes." I take a deep breath in, exhale it out, but nothing changes. I continue to obsess. I take another breath. Nothing. A third. And this time, as I exhale, I feel the anxiety shift a little. So I keep breathing, a little deeper each time, until the panic lessens enough that I'm able to leave the studio at the end of class without accosting the teacher.

The next day I leave my apartment, lock the door, and count the fifty-six steps to the bottom, as I always do. I turn around to go back up, but for some reason I stop, sit down on the bottom stair, and wait. I want to leave the building and get on with my day, but I know I can't, not until I climb back up those stairs and repeat the ritual four times. But I don't. Instead, I sit there and watch my anxiety rise. I feel its energy—jittery, fluttery, hot, tingling, electric, and uncomfortable—and I remember what the teacher had said the day before. "Breathe and everything changes." So I breathe, but nothing changes. I keep breathing, and the anxiety gets worse. I keep breathing, and finally, I feel a shift. The sensations lessen, and the panic subsides. After a while I stand up and straighten out my clothes. I glance back up the stairs, take another deep breath, and then turn toward the front door and leave the building.

TEACHINGS FROM THE STAIRWELL
THERAPY, PRANAYAMA, AND TRAUMA

In therapy, Norman helped me connect the dots between my OCD behaviors and my childhood trauma, which I wasn't even aware I had. He helped me understand that all people experience some degree of trauma in their lives but not always in the same way. An event that seems like no big deal to one person can leave someone else unable to function. Many of us, in fact, tend to minimize our traumas because they don't seem, well, traumatic enough. We tend to think what others have experienced is far worse than what we've been through. And anyway, we're fine now.

Trauma can be a one-time event, or it can be ongoing. Developmental trauma, which most experts agree is the hardest to treat, involves situations that happen in our childhood, events we felt powerless to stop, such as rejection, abandonment, bullying, the death of a loved one, and any kind of abuse—physical, emotional, or sexual. Shock trauma happens after events occur unexpectedly that we were not prepared for, such as rape and other kinds of violence, having someone die unexpectedly, being in a car accident, discovering a partner is having an affair, or losing a child.

Working with Norman helped me *admit* my trauma, but doing yoga helped me *access* it in ways that years of talking about it never could. Why? Because trauma lives in the body—and cannot be reasoned away. "Our issues live in our tissues," as yogis are fond of saying, and they are kept alive by our obsessive thoughts. While we're busy in therapy trying to understand—or rationalize—those issues and learning tools to manage them, our bodies are busy holding on tightly to the "story," which can include the loss of our five-year-old self, the heartbreak of our thirteen-year-old self, the righteous indignation of our twenty-two-year-old self, or myriad other experiences. Our bodies keep everything we've ever repressed, locked away in our muscles, joints, and cellular tissue. Our bodies remember everything.

Even though trauma is a *physiological* response to a horrific event or perceived threat, the mind has to be engaged in the process if healing is to happen. You need to see and feel what's coming up, as it's happening, and commit to staying present and investigating your narrative, your internal experience—without judgment. In other words, you need to employ both the mind *and* the body in concert. Otherwise, you're just churning up energy and not changing anything, maybe even making things worse. How does trauma get lodged in the body in the first place, and what happens to us when it does? How would a suggestion such as "breathe and everything changes" make such a profound difference? Let's start with a little physiology lesson.

TRAUMA: THE INSIDE SCOOP

First of all, we are all hardwired to survive. Anything that compromises your experience of safety and security triggers a biochemical reaction, a "Danger!" alert that throws your system into action without you ever having to think about it. So you perceive a threat. Instantaneously, the brain sends a message to the thalamus, a small organ within the brain that determines where the threat is coming from and then, not really knowing whether the event is hostile or not, passes the information on to the amygdala, which signals the hypothalamus to initiate the fight-flight-freeze-fold response, just in case. The fight-flight-freeze-fold response begins as the sympathetic nervous system goes into high gear, along with the adrenal-cortical system, activating a whole host of stress hormones, including cortisol, epinephrine, and norepinephrine. Everything critical to your survival is alerted. The increase of hormones blocks pain and decreases inflammation; cortisol releases sugar as fuel into the bloodstream so you can think and move faster; heart rate and blood pressure rise; your pupils dilate; and your blood vessels constrict, shunting blood to the major muscle groups so you have more strength and power. Everything that is not essential to your survival shuts down: the digestive, reproductive, immune, and cellular-repair systems. You are now ready to either stay and confront the threat (fight) or get the hell out of there (flight). The freeze-or-fold response causes you to either dissociate in any number of ways (freeze) or collapse or capitulate (fold).

All this fight, flight, freeze, or fold business is normal, an important part of our survival—just like it is for animals in the wild—but it's designed to be short-lived. In the wild, as soon as the threat passes, an animal's safety depends on her ability to put that experience behind her and get on with her day. She will quite literally shake it off. Our nervous system is wired to do the same thing. The threat passes, and we "shake it off" by crying, trembling, or screaming—anything we can do to discharge the energy and release the tension from the body. Then the parasympathetic nervous system (the system involved in resting and digesting) takes over, restoring the ease and balance that is the body's natural state. The body and the mind need time to "digest" what just happened, so, depending on what you've experienced, it may take a while for everything to get back to normal, including your heart rate, blood pressure, and various systems in the body. When it does, you can also get on with your day. However, the *residue* of that event never goes away; it gets stored in your cellular memory and becomes a part of your history, the stories you tell yourself.

If you don't shake it off—that is, if you fail to acknowledge and process the emotional fallout—the rest-and-digest process (the body's "rinse cycle") gets interrupted. Denying or bypassing negative thoughts and feelings or avoiding situations that remind you of the original trauma will prevent the body from being able to rid itself of the trauma you initially experienced. At that point, those undigested emotions (anger, fear, shame) become entangled in the residue and indistinguishable from the original event.

When all this happens, any new situation you experience that's even mildly uncomfortable or feels unsafe produces a biochemical reaction akin to the first trauma. Before you're even aware of what's happening, your brain has checked out and time traveled back to the original stressor. Your nervous system thinks the original event is happening all over again and goes on high-alert—or on shut-down mode. All the repressed emotion that got buried after the initial event is energy, just like everything in the body. Its chaotic vibration lies dormant until the moment it gets activated. Suddenly the mildly uncomfortable situation has become an emotionally heightened one. To feel better, to shift the energy, you may find yourself becoming reactive. This can include getting into arguments or fights, or you may shut down, space out, and not feel a thing. When this happens, you might turn to food, sex, drugs, alcohol, and other addictions—anything that will help you feel better without having to actually *feel* anything.

All the undigested emotions and their associated energy—the fear, anger, rage, shame, or helplessness—live on in the body, hidden away, and can manifest as muscular tension. Over time, the tension becomes so familiar, so predictable, that it feels perfectly normal and safe. What's not normal or safe, of course, are the emotions that lie trapped beneath the tension.

THE ROLE YOGA PLAYS

Remember, trauma experts say that we must employ the mind *and* the body in order to release tension and heal from trauma. Yoga, as a body-based meditation practice, does that by creating space and freedom in the body, mind, and heart through asana, pranayama, and meditation. By doing asana, the body identifies long-held tension—or stored energy—in the musculature and can bring it to light,

which may not always feel that great. But that's not all. Old, forgotten emotions, embedded in those muscles, often come along for the ride, demanding to be seen and felt by the mind and the heart. That doesn't always feel so great, either. Nonetheless, seeing and acknowledging the energy is the only way to get it unstuck and usher it out of the body.

Moving the body releases tension. Being physical unties knots. Engaging the mind gives us context and allows us to investigate what's bubbling up. When we enter into a pose, we scan the body for sensation and then breathe and observe. What are we feeling? Physically? Emotionally? Where does the tension lie? Where are the areas of contraction? Focusing on the breath, we can see the places in the body that feel stuck, that need physical release and emotional reconciliation. What lives there? What's the story? Breathing into sensation quiets the reactive manomaya kosha—the monkey mind that can't seem to leave things alone—and engages the heart. The heart center—also called the wisdom mind, or vijnanamaya kosha—invites us to notice our experiences *as they are happening* without judgment and without the intrusion of painful memories.

The monkey mind definitely gets us in trouble and can keep us stuck. *Yoga chitta vritti nirodhah.* That oft-quoted passage in the Yoga Sutras means yoga is the taming of the fluctuations or chatter (*vrittis*) of the mind (*chitta*). Think of vrittis as the endless loop of stories you tell yourself, the ones that keep you tethered to a "less-than" or "I'm not worthy" script that plays on repeat in your mind. Getting caught up in that narrative causes us to further contract around our pain, and our inner and outer worlds become smaller and narrower. We live in our shadow, and we see the world through that lens. By calming or silencing the mind even for a breath or two, we can find the space and freedom we need to heal.

When I was in Downward-Facing Dog that day in yoga class, my mind kept reeling from my inability to "even out" the sensation I felt after my teacher bumped my foot. The more I dwelt on the event, the more anxious I became. Then he said, "Breathe and everything changes." Those four words brought my obsessive thinking to a standstill and moved my attention into my body. At first, nothing happened. Or so I thought. But what was really happening was exactly what needed

to happen to start the process. My mind needed to notice what my body was feeling. Sure, I kept fixating, but I didn't walk away. I continued to breathe, and my mind continued to investigate, until a little opening appeared, an almost imperceptible release of tension. As I kept breathing, that opening expanded, and by the end of class, I felt free enough, composed enough, to walk out—without indulging the compulsion.

Breathe and everything changes. Find the breath, and you find the mind. Find the breath, and the mind returns to the present, which is the only place breath happens. Find the mind, and it can direct the breath to those places in the body that need the most attention. Working with this simple teaching can decrease the tension we hold in the body and the mind dramatically. It yields a physiological response that can dampen down fight-flight-freeze-fold reactivity and encourage rest-and-digest, wait-and-see receptivity, which can break the cycle of ritualized behavior. Beyond that, it invites us to hit the pause button. To wait. To notice. Yogis love to go there, exhaling into that pause, the gap before the inhalation comes again, where we move from doing to simply being, from obsession to reflection. The gap where true liberation happens—liberation from doubts, fears, memories, and traumas—even if only for a single moment.

But that day on the stairs, I was just happy that yoga released the tension in my body enough to decrease my anxiety, and help me be less reactive and more present. I'm not suggesting that my OCD was cured, not by a long shot. OCD is a complex condition that is different for everyone. But connecting with the breath gave me one essential tool I could always use so that, in time and with practice, I could be liberated from the bonds of my compulsive behaviors. But I certainly wasn't ready for too much self-reflection or self-reveal. Not yet.

Yoga's job is to show you what's *actually* happening—not what the mind *thinks* is happening or *wants* to happen. Yoga exposes truth; it allows the stories buried deep within the body to emerge out of the tension you've released and into the open spaces you've created. But, here's the thing: only if you are open to receiving them. And that's not easy.

Whenever we move, breathe, stretch, activate the ego, and push ourselves to our personal edge, big feelings can come up on the mat. We might get anxious, fidgety, look around, nod off, make jokes—anything to shift or change the sensation. I was a master at that. In life, when we get uncomfortable or big emotions arise, we can turn to food, drugs and alcohol, sex, or even shopping or TV watching to change or alter those feelings. I was a master at that too. On the yoga mat, we don't have access to our go-to distractions; all we have are our senses, our mind, and our breath. So it's important to allow the thoughts, the feelings, and the fantasies to arise—without judgment. We have to look at how the mind keeps us distracted or even disempowered. This is essential to our healing because however we deal with discomfort on the mat mirrors how we behave when we're challenged in life.

Yoga is not a get-fixed-quick scheme. In fact, in the Yoga Sutras, Patanjali says you must commit to diligent, disciplined practice (*abhyasa*) to keep the mind coming back to the present moment. In other words, in order for yoga to help, you must do the work! You must be willing to bring everything to the surface and investigate it. But, he says, don't get consumed by what you discover.

Loosen the grip (*vairagya*) it has on you, relax the identity it gives you, and simply let it be. Can you observe something as it presents itself and not get caught up in it?

That commitment to practice and surrender (abhyasa and vairagya) is hard to do because, as I learned, we can get unwittingly "addicted" to our tension, limiting beliefs, and disconnected feelings, all of which create a biochemical response that becomes all too familiar, predictable, and oddly comforting. None of this happens consciously of course. Our subconscious defaults to what it knows and encourages the sensation to surface that will keep us on high alert—more tension, defensiveness, numbing out—so we can never be hurt or taken by surprise again.

Yet commit we must because the inability to heal fractures created by the effects of trauma and unprocessed emotions can only lead to more suffering and a deeper split within ourselves. Without yoga or other trauma-informed practices to help us feel whole again, we have no self-awareness, no self-love; without self-understanding, there can be no collective understanding, no sense of union. And we all suffer. To alleviate that suffering, we must come into union within ourselves, body and mind. This is the work of yoga. This is the evolution of the soul. This is the pathway to freedom.

5

BREAK ON THROUGH TO THE OTHER SIDE

SOMETIME IN 1991 I got it in my head that I wanted to move to Los Angeles.

I've had a romantic notion of Southern California for as long as I can remember. Probably because I was raised on the East Coast. Its no-nonsense, hard-edged, straightforward culture—which I found exhilarating and, at times, absolutely exhausting—was the exact opposite of the progressive, open, and alternative-everything lifestyle I imagined on the West Coast. I had no clue whether any of my perceptions were actually true; I just knew I wanted what Led Zeppelin sang about in "Going to California." I'd hang in Central Park, get stoned, and listen to Robert Plant describe the "aching" in his heart and the girl with "flowers in her hair," and I would think, *That's me! I have an aching! I'd wear flowers!*

I couldn't get the image of California tranquility out of my mind. I was tired of New York. Tired of nightclubs. Tired of feeling unsettled about my future. Perhaps a change of scenery would give me the inspiration I needed to help me understand my purpose.

LA was hardly the picture Robert Plant painted. (I'm pretty sure he was singing about San Francisco. Oh well.) As the heart of the entertainment industry, LA can be superficial and egocentric, a place that raises hopes and shatters dreams.

But it's also a hotbed of alternative health and healing practices. Everything new, experiential, and far-out can still be found there. It was so different than New York in that way, and I took every opportunity to expand my awareness.

But at the beginning, I was lonely. I'd wake up every day in the small, furnished room I rented in Los Feliz to the smell of piss and shit wafting in on the morning breeze from the narrow dog run—the view from my only window. Confused about next steps and far away from my family and friends, I felt my anxiety rise up more frequently. My old OCD behaviors were tugging at me, promising relief. Six months after moving from one coast to the other, I hadn't found a yoga studio yet, nor did I have the money to go. So I wasn't practicing and, as a result, I had fallen into some old habits. I wasn't drinking or doing drugs, but I was being less than honest in my relationships yet again. I was seeing a man, an actor, whom I had known since I was young. We were very into one another, and we spent a lot of time together. Problem was, I was also into my boyfriend back in New York. I felt awful about being so deceptive, but I felt worse about being alone. I knew that I needed to find a yoga class soon, otherwise I'd end up hurting them both and acting out in other ways as well.

My LA boyfriend gave me a book by Jiddu Krishnamurti, an Indian philosopher who wrote about the need for a revolution of the psyche and the "spiritual freedom" that follows. I read it cover to cover. Krishnamurti's philosophy on consciousness and the necessity to "change the thinker" attracted me and in my quest to find more teachings like that, I stumbled upon Paramahansa Yogananda's book *An Autobiography of a Yogi*. The book was a bit too mythological for my tastes, but still, I was curious to know more, so I decided to pay a visit to the Self-Realization Fellowship (SRF), the center for all things Yogananda, in Pacific Palisades. Wandering through a pristine park on the grounds, I felt a deep sense of contentment wash over me.

I walked through the doors of SRF and struck up a conversation with the woman behind the counter. She told me her daughter went to YogaWorks, which was in Santa Monica, and loved it. I drove up the street looking for it and spotted the sign on the second floor of a building on the corner of 15th and Montana. That turn up the driveway would be the turn that changed the direction of my whole life.

I parked the car and entered the small studio. There were two practice rooms and two waiting rooms in between. I looked around at the familiar books on the shelves and pictures on the wall and inhaled the wafting scent of Nag Champa incense, a yoga studio staple. I didn't feel as out of place as I had the first time I went to Integral Yoga, but the scene in LA was definitely different, and I clearly stood out with my combat boots, heavy black eyeliner, and big hair. It felt more like a club than the yoga studios I was used to back in New York. In the lounge, the music had a high energy, techno New Age sound. Sprawled out on the couches and floor were young, gorgeous-looking people decked out in brightly colored, skintight Lycra leggings with bra tops or shorts with expensive-looking T-shirts. And from what I could tell, no one seemed to be wearing any underwear! I reached around to my own backside and touched the lines of my granny panties under my thick sweats. I felt awkward and out of place. A woman in a handstand against the wall turned her head toward me and told me I needed to take off my shoes; wow, was I ever embarrassed for making such a rookie mistake.

After I removed my boots and placed them in the shoe racks next to endless rows of flip-flops, Birkenstocks, and Ugg boots, I went back into the lounge area and saw a petite woman sitting on a couch, with long, dark braids, olive skin, and huge teal eyes. She was wearing a pale-green tank top and matching leggings, the bottoms pulled halfway over each foot. She was chatting with the people around her; her direct, nasal voice had an air of command, and she seemed to both know and be interested in everyone around her. I was drawn to her unusual beauty and sat down nearby, quietly taking in the scene and this tiny queen holding court. I had no idea that she was Maty Ezraty, the cofounder of YogaWorks and that she would one day become my mentor.

Maty started YogaWorks with her then-husband Chuck Miller. It was the most eclectic yoga studio I had ever been to. You could take Iyengar or Kundalini yoga classes if you wanted to; they offered Ashtanga and Power Yoga too; restorative practices, and even prenatal and a special Mommy-and-Me hour. Pretty much every kind of yoga practice was offered, and the desk staff encouraged the students to explore the diverse styles. Most yoga studios at that time were dedicated to a single form of yoga and were more traditional and austere. YogaWorks was social and friendly, and Maty encouraged this sense of community.

I took a job volunteering there because I couldn't afford classes. For every hour I stuffed envelopes or made calls, I would get a free class. Eventually, I was volunteering so much that Maty gave me a job as a receptionist. For the first time since I was seventeen, I wasn't working in a restaurant or a bar, so I had to figure out how to pay my bills on a low hourly wage. The perk was that I could take as many classes and workshops as I wanted—for free. I took advantage of it. I practiced at least twice a day—Ashtanga with Chuck every morning and then, in the evening after my shift, with whoever else was on the schedule. It didn't really matter, I loved it all.

Even though I was immersed in the physical practice, I still secretly rolled my eyes when teachers chanted and shared their philosophical interpretations. Sometimes Chuck would sit down next to me, after adjusting me in a pose, and go on and on about the deeper meaning of the posture, or some esoterica he thought I needed to understand. I would nod my head, but I had no idea what he was talking about. I still cringed a little when I heard "Spirit," "Divine," "Consciousness," or any other word people around me used to describe God. My distrust in the spiritual realm ran deep. It all smacked of religion, and I didn't want any part of it. Nonetheless, I recognized my resistance and could acknowledge (at least to myself) that I really was looking for, and craving, more meaning in my life.

Billy's words would often rise to the surface, reminding me to see the God within. I wanted to, but none of what I was learning fully landed in my heart the way I hoped it would. For Billy, love was inclusive; God resided within all. It made sense to me intellectually, but I heartily rejected any kind of relationship with any kind of God, especially the one I had implored for years not to hurt the people I loved. This push-pull confused me. I wanted connection, and, at the same time, I rejected connection. I'd sometimes look around the room during meditation and see the other students, who all looked so beautiful, their eyes lifting skyward, bliss etched into their faces. I felt jealous and inept. I couldn't get still enough to experience the Divine speaking to me and through me from within, as I was told would happen if I'd just shut my friggin' eyes and try. Spirituality eluded me—*What if I don't have a God within me?*—and I felt deeply stuck in my own story of resistance.

After months of working behind the desk, I decided to take Bryan Kest's Power Yoga class. I had heard of Bryan but hadn't seen or met him yet. A few days before, as I was coming back to the studio after lunch, I saw this unbelievably handsome guy sitting on the hood of my blue Geo Metro, talking to a group of people who were hanging on his every word. He had long curly hair, was shirtless and barefoot, clad only in a pair of denim shorts. *What the hell? Get your ass off my car!* He glanced over at me and, I had to admit, my heart skipped a beat. I thought, *Uh-oh. I think that's my new boyfriend.* He turned away and then did a quick double take, our eyes catching. I held his gaze, and rocking my best New York aloof-and-unavailable response, I looked away without smiling and turned into the studio. *Yup,* I thought, *He's mine.*

I would find out soon enough that the man on my car was indeed Bryan Kest, arguably the most popular teacher in LA, if not the nation. Power Yoga, a highly physical offshoot of Ashtanga yoga, one that blended various styles of yoga asana and philosophy into a single class, was *the* practice to do in the '90s and Bryan's classes were packed—hot, sweaty, and filled with gym folk, moms and pops, rock and movie stars, and hard-core yogis. He attracted an eclectic group of people, young and old, who shared a few particular traits—a love of sweat, hard work, and a certain enthusiasm that definitely intrigued me.

The first time I took Bryan's class, sweat literally poured off me—onto my mat, the floor, and the mats next to me. I understood why everyone was wearing skintight Lycra and why sweats and T-shirts didn't belong in Power Yoga. I spent most of the class untangling myself from my soaking wet T-shirt. In another week or so, my mom would save me from myself and send a box of bright-colored leggings and sports bras from TJ Maxx—and even include a thong! I just love my mother.

Bryan taught class differently than anyone I had ever experienced before. There was no commanding silence when you entered the room. Instead, everyone was chatty, laughing, and loud. There was no New Age music to accompany class. It was just Bryan's Detroit-laced accent waxing poetic; his words were no-nonsense, demanding, and intense. He brought his entire personality into the room and shared his experience of yoga straight from the heart. He articulated traditional concepts in a way that made them accessible. He dropped the F-bomb, was motivational, and alluded to sex and heartbreak and loss and hope and to all things human. Bryan was very much of this world, and because of his authenticity, he attracted people who probably wouldn't have shown up to a conventional yoga class. Bryan was changing the face of contemporary yoga and speaking to the hearts of ordinary people who wanted transformation—and strong abs!

It was a scene, and I loved it. His classes were powerful and empowering.

Eventually, Bryan and I fell in love and became a couple, albeit briefly. Although I do not necessarily recommend dating your yoga teacher for many, many reasons, Bryan inspired me to teach and helped me find my own voice in the process. Once again, our angels are everywhere, and Bryan Kest absolutely proved to be a potent one in my life.

It was also in Bryan's class that I had my first true emotional breakthrough, which caused long-held and deeply suppressed emotions, lodged within my flesh, to surface, cracking the armor that had formed in my body and most certainly around my heart. Here's what happened.

▼

On this particular day, I'm practicing next to a beautiful young woman. She's strong, lithe, and focused. She floats through her practice so naturally that I become obsessed with her. *If I were as thin as she is, I'd feel less clunky. She has really nice leggings; she's probably wealthy. Figures. Is that her real nose? Doubt it. No way are those her boobs. No way.* Every time Bryan adjusts her, I bristle. *Did she just giggle when he touched her? Not cool.* I'm probably "in my ego," as Bryan and other teachers like to say, but honestly, I don't even know what that means. And I don't care. I remember Chuck often reminding us not to "identify with the voices in your head." I don't know what that means either. All I know is that Bryan seems to be making yet another unnecessary adjustment on this woman, who I decide is shallow, spoiled, and fake. I am now referring to her as "LA Girl." I know I'm being judgy, but I don't care about that, either.

I hear Bryan tell us to come into Pigeon Pose, and I feel a momentary relief knowing that we are heading to the floor to do more passive poses. Pigeon is a particularly intense hip opener, one that Bryan always enjoys having us hold for an ungodly amount of time. Because of my flexibility, that has never bothered me. Pigeon is more of a resting pose for me, and I like hanging out in it, indulging in the stretch. Bryan often takes the opportunity to speak to the deeper aspects of yoga such as acceptance, equanimity, unity, forgiveness, and love—and I often take the opportunity to tune him out. So, as usual, he's yammering on, and I'm zoning out, thinking about everything except what he's saying or what's happening in my body. I have a hard time settling—the sensation in my hip is uncomfortable. I don't get it. I usually can just relax, even fall asleep, but on this day my body aches in areas I've never felt before. *Why the hell am I so tight today?* I move my body to find a more comfortable position.

My mind wanders to what Bryan and I might do after class. *Hike? Eat? Hump?* That last thought makes me smile, and the sensation in my hip eases a bit. Then I wonder whether or not I could teach my cat Zooey to walk on a leash so I could take him everywhere I went. *That would be amazing.* I smile again at the thought and chuckle to myself, my body relaxing a little more. My mind then drifts to how I'm going to get the money to buy a plane ticket home for Christmas. *Maybe I can pick up some extra shifts?* The pain comes back, and I change my position slightly once again. My mind continues to jump from thought to thought as I reflect on everything from LA Girl, who I'm sure is after my boyfriend, to my family, my relationships, and my future. It seems endless. The whole time I keep shifting in my posture trying to find a place of comfort in my body. It's not happening, and I feel myself becoming more agitated. LA Girl is breathing deeply and loudly. The intensity of her ujjayi pranayama practice is not necessary at this point in the class, and I keep sending her sharp looks hoping she'll get the hint and tone it down. I fidget some more. I keep glancing around the room, discreetly checking out the people around me, wondering a bit about their lives. "Breathe!" Bryan commands. "Keep your attention on your own mat!" and I put my head back down, embarrassed, convinced he is speaking only to me.

Breathing into my smelly mat, my head resting in a pool of my sweat, I wonder how much longer he plans to make us hold this fucking pose. LA Girl starts to quietly moan. Christ, I think, just fucking be quiet! By now I'm truly annoyed, and I feel my exasperation toward her, toward Bryan, toward everyone and everything increase with every inhale and exhale. More low moans and groans come from the students around me as Bryan continues to drone on and my restlessness and annoyance continue to increase.

I lie there hating the whole world and everyone in it, including myself. My body feels contracted; the pain in my hip radiates down my leg. Suddenly, out of nowhere, I inhale sharply, and a high, awkward gulping sound rises up from deep within me, as though my breath had gotten caught in the back of my throat. It takes me by surprise, and I glance around to see if anyone else noticed. Once again, Bryan says randomly to the room, "Breathe!" I do, and the sound comes through me again. Lying there, eyes wide open, I feel my whole body begin to tremble. I look at my fingers, and they won't stay still. A new layer of sweat forms on my brow, although it's no longer scorching hot in the room. My heart is beating fast, and I can feel heat rise in my chest. A heaviness settles behind my eyes, my nose and lips become thick and full, and I know my face is red. I am holding my breath. I realize then, with true alarm, that I am about to cry. What the fuck? I can feel my whole body freeze up, my breath lodged somewhere in my chest. I am embarrassed and anxious. I do not want to cry here. I do not want to cry at all! I try to think about something else. *Hike. Sex. Christmas. Ticket. Cat.* Nothing helps. A tear falls onto my mat. I stare at it. Another one falls. Then another. Finally, I force myself to get out of the pose and out of the room. I keep my head down, hoping not to slip on the puddles of sweat between me and the door. I burst into tears before I make it to the bathroom.

In the stall, I heave. Tears pouring from my eyes, deep, animal sounds coming from inside me. I don't get it. Everything in my life is fine; it really is. I have a job I enjoy, a boyfriend I'm into, a practice I love.

Why am I so suddenly, so unexpectedly, emotional? This isn't like me at all. I'm a lot of things, but I'm not a crier; I take pride in not being "like a girl." Growing up in a family of only brothers, male cousins, and uncles, I learned early that crying got you nowhere, and if I wanted to play with the "big boys," I had to learn to "take it like a man." So I rarely cried. Whenever I feel emotional, my first instinct has always been to hold my breath or to lash out. I remember Norman saying that not crying was a part of my dissociation, that I shoved my feelings down deep inside and made myself numb out so I wouldn't feel anything. Feelings weren't safe for me. They were chaotic and scary, and so to avoid them, I repressed them. Raging, something I did frequently, especially in the face of injustice, could also make me "feel better," temporarily. It's not that I *never* cried, it's just that when I did, I had a good reason to. But never like this! This inexplicably came out of nowhere and felt endless—and somehow ancient.

I slide down the wall and hug my knees into my chest. My body convulses as a lifetime of tears pour out of me, and I have no idea if they'll ever stop. My chest feels hot, my heart beats fast, my jaw is tight, and I'm tingling from head to toe.

I instinctively keep shaking out my arms and hands because they feel numb and thick. I say out loud, over and over, "What the fuck? What the fuck?"

I keep glancing at the door, praying no one will come in and find me like this. I feel so ashamed. There seems to be a bottomless well of tears in my body, and I am literally trying to shake them out of me.

The tears finally stop, though my body is still buzzing and trembly. I get up and, without looking in the mirror, splash water on my face, welcoming the cool of the liquid on my skin. I take a few deep breaths, and with my arms and legs quivering slightly, make my way back to class, avoiding Bryan's eyes, and sit down on the floor. By then everyone has settled into Pigeon Pose on the second side. I can still hear random low moans and groans and the occasional sniffle from the students nearby. I wonder if they've been crying too. Is this a thing?

I move into the pose and lie there breathing, feeling spent and confused. I recite my mantra "Breathe and everything changes" and let the deep breaths come in and out of me, feeling my heart slow down little by little. I notice the sensation in my hip and place my awareness on the exact spot where the feeling is most intense. Anxiety wells up in me once again, but I continue breathing into that one spot, my attention fixed, my breath deep. *You're okay,* I tell myself. *Breathe into it.*

I find myself concentrating on every word Bryan says, at first as a means of distraction. He's talking about the ways in which we heal. As his words find their way to me—something about acceptance, compassion, and trust—I bite down on my lip, but my tears come again and the heat in my left hip intensifies. He reminds us to focus on the sensation, so I bring all of my attention to what I'm feeling and try to relax into it. The sensation is thick, sharp, and stabby, and it's beginning to throb. Behind my closed eyes, I see the color red. I've never seen colors before when I practice. Other images begin to appear. I see my childhood house, a small brick colonial set back off the street, a large oak tree off to the side. I enter the house, go up the stairs, the thick green shag carpet soft on my feet. I'm standing in the hallway where I used to sleep when guests were over, and my own room was being used. I see my young self lying on the floor, on my belly, my nightgown pulled up over my hips. I see a young man in his underwear lying next to me, giggling, a finger to his lips, telling me to *shhh* . . .

My body starts to shake again as I come back into the present, and I feel myself contract, my muscles tighten. I'm afraid I might get sick. I take another breath, relax, and as the shaking continues, the tears I couldn't cry at six come pouring out of me. Images from that night keep surfacing. I don't stop them, even as my brain keeps trying to grab other thoughts. *Plane ticket home! Cat on leash!* I gently remind myself to breathe.

I hear Bryan say, "Remain equanimous to your experience. Stay in your body and be present to whatever rises. Try not to judge it. Just witness what comes up . . ."

Stay in my body? Be present? I remember that feeling of floating above myself, watching my six-year-old body being touched, as though it were happening to someone else. I feel so sad for that poor girl lying there frozen, her eyes wide open, his hands now between her legs. I think to myself, *My body has never been safe. How can I be present? If I'm present, I have to do something, and I can't. I am frozen!*

I then realize that I am frozen—even in this moment. I don't think I could move or get out of the pose even if I wanted to. I tell myself to shift a bit, and I feel instant relief. I *can* move. I *can* get away now, if I need to. I start discreetly tapping on the floor in patterns of four.

Bryan moves through the room reminding us that our bodies have wisdom. Let your body speak to you, he says.

I stop patterning and take another breath. That's exactly what is happening, I think. My body is speaking to me. It wants to tell its story. Long-held feelings and memories buried deep in my cells begin to surface. For the first time in my life, I sense that there is an intelligence within my body that craves expression.

Anxiety, a feeling so familiar to me, keeps clawing its way to the top of my awareness. Although I want to stay present, another part of me would rather dissociate. *No,* I think. *Stay with this, Seane. Breathe into this. Don't run, please! What does your body want to say?*

As my body continues to quiver and pulse, I give myself full permission, even in this public space, to sob into the towel on my mat. Great heaves move through me like they did in the bathroom only a few minutes before. I'm both mortified and relieved. The tears are cleansing my body of what seems like lifetimes of anger and pain and grief I didn't even know were there.

Bryan invites us to come out of the pose, and as I sit up and release my leg, energy rushes into my pelvis and hip joint. I gently shake them out. It's such a relief. I can feel the prana, the life-force, activated in my legs, and they feel light and open. I blow my nose into the bottom of my T-shirt. I don't look around. I don't want to catch anyone's eye.

Bryan tells us to straighten both legs in front of us, inhale our arms overhead, and fold forward, grabbing hold of our legs, feet, or big toes. I follow his instructions, resting my chest on my thighs and grabbing onto my toes. I turn my head to the side and rest there, letting my body surrender to this deep stretch.

Bryan comes over to me, places both hands onto my lower back and gently presses me deeper into the pose. The scream I wanted to make twenty years earlier rushes to the top of my throat but stops short of pouring out of me. I push my back up against him in resistance. I don't want his hands there. I don't want to be touched, but I don't know how to ask him to stop. *Doesn't he know better? Am I overreacting? What if I hurt his feelings?* I freeze. When have I had those thoughts before? I again see the little me lying on her belly, his large hand on the small of her back, holding her in place. My body is pissed. I quickly shift under the weight of Bryan's hands, and, perhaps picking up on an unspoken signal, he moves away. I exhale with my whole body; the anger softens.

Sitting on the stage at the front of the room, Bryan speaks of the fragility of the human experience, the challenges we all face, and the ways in which these challenges expand our perspective and open our hearts . . . if we allow them to. He talks about Spirit, self-love, equanimity, and the importance of letting the emotions "trapped" inside of us out so they no longer have power. He speaks of vulnerability, of surrender, and of acceptance.

I hear Billy's words coming through Bryan. But I'm not just *hearing* them this time, I'm *feeling* them—on every level—and they make perfect sense. Life happens; it just does. The miracles are in the process, the journey, not the destination itself. How someone evolves, I remember Billy telling me, was between each being and the God of their understanding. Sometimes it's messy, always it's perfect, and each experience, every moment, opens us to love. Is that what's happening to me? Am I opening to love? Then why does it hurt so much?

My body trembles, absorbing and rejecting each word Bryan utters. I can feel this internal struggle between surrender and defiance. My ego pushes back. *It's all right,* I think. *Something is happening. You are okay,* I tell myself again. *Your body has something to say. Just be present.*

Bryan then says something about forgiveness.

My body tightens and rage rips through me once again. *Forgiveness? Are you fucking kidding me? Fuck you!* I screamed in my head, silently addressing my molester. I am surprised by the intensity of my reaction. My anger scares me, and I start to shake again. How deep does this rage go? Then, as though reading my mind, Bryan suggests to the class: "Start with yourself. Forgive yourself for thinking you should have known better."

Forgive myself? My whole body releases into the floor. The tension melts away. My eyes open, and I stare at the floor in front of me. I exhale fully.

I let myself see the beautiful girl that I had been, and I feel an enormous amount of compassion for this bright and sensitive soul. I realize how deeply her story lives in my body, and I see all the ways in which I have managed to control the physical and emotional discomfort that has never really gone away. I knew I was angry, deeply angry, and that this anger has been with me a long, long time. I also knew that I have avoided this anger, and the grief beneath it, by running away from it in different ways over all these years. In that moment, I realize that by running away from my grief, I have also abandoned the tenderest parts of myself and left her, my little self, behind. I make a silent commitment to myself that I will never abandon or betray the little girl within me again. I know I have a lot of work ahead of me, but I want to protect her and give her a voice and hear what she needs to say. "I am so sorry," I say to her and to my body. I have learned how to cope, but now I want to learn how to heal. I haven't a clue how to do that, but I know that I must, and I will. "I am so sorry," I repeat again and again.

Bryan then asks us to lie on our back for Savasana. I lie flat and settle myself onto the ground, feeling the support of the earth beneath me. I feel a deep sense of relief, as though pounds of tension have melted from my body. I can still hear Bryan speaking somewhere in the room, saying something about surrendering to the Mother. I think of my own mother and feel a rush of love move through me. *I will love myself the way that my mother loves me,* I think to myself. Purely and unconditionally. I imagine my mom embracing me, as I embrace my little self. I then imagine all of us enveloped by an infinite feminine force. Slowly, in this pocket of love, my consciousness drifts further and further away. I feel the fog lift; every word Bryan has said makes sense and spoke directly to my soul. It was as though he has been speaking to my heart in a language that I had always known, but somehow forgotten. It felt embodied. He didn't say anything new. Billy had said it. David and Sharon had said it, the rabbi-guru in New York had said it, Krishnamurti and Yogananda had said it, Maty and Chuck, and all the teachers I had practiced with had said it too, in their own way. Nothing had really changed . . . except me. Something has shifted, my awareness has expanded, and I slowly drift off into something like sleep.

Soon I hear Bryan invite us to roll onto our side and sit up for meditation. I feel dazed, but absolutely fine. Instead of squirming and feeling impatient as I usually do in meditation, I sit tall and still. I've never felt so open or connected to myself before. I feel free—or maybe it's whole? Whatever it is, it's beautiful. I listen to my heart beat, turn my attention inside, and feel utterly grounded in the moment. I don't want to move and am so happy to be with myself in this way, in silence.

Bryan keeps us there for quite a while, and I bask in the stillness I feel. I'm aware I've gone through quite a metamorphosis. Not quite like the caterpillar becoming the butterfly, more like how it becomes the pupa first. Messy and emulsified, but rich with possibility. I smile at that thought. I suspect I should feel embarrassed by what happened. I know I drew attention to myself, but I couldn't care less. I feel at peace.

In time, Bryan instructs us to place our hands back into prayer and then says, "Namaste." We all say it back, and this time I really mean it. I bow my head, open my eyes, and glance sheepishly toward LA Girl, who is staring right at me. She is wide-eyed and concerned. She leans forward, touches my arm gently, and asks if I'm okay. I take in this young woman and think of all the assumptions I made, and ways I had judged her, and what her presence inspired in me that day. I'm sure I must look like a hot mess between the sweat, the tears, and the snot. I go to speak, but no words come out. I suddenly burst out laughing. She looks at me even more curiously, but then smiles, too. I throw my arms around her and pull her in for a hug. She hugs me back in surprise and then starts to laugh as well. After a bit she asks, "What happened?"

I pull back to look at her and say, "I have no fucking clue. But whatever that was? It was good. Really good."

TEACHINGS FROM THE MAT
MIND-BODY CONNECTION, SHADOW WORK, AND RELEASE

I can't say that I welcomed the experience that day on the mat (or in the bathroom), but because I had done plenty of trauma therapy with Norman and years of embodied work through yoga, I chose to stay with it, breathe into it, and bear witness to what was coming up. Make no mistake, though, I was confronting and releasing some long-held trauma from my body; I got triggered, tried to dissociate, and at times came close to being re-traumatized—and that can be pretty scary. I *was* scared, but not so overwhelmed that I felt unsafe or that I lacked the tools I needed to take care of myself.

If you are dealing with trauma or have a sense that painful narratives remain buried in your cells, it's important to take things slow. Here are a few things to keep in mind.

First, talk therapy, in conjunction with a body-based practice, such as yoga, can be extremely helpful in trying to unpack and release trauma and unprocessed emotions.

Second, if you practice yoga, you can always come out of a pose, at any time, if the sensations get too intense or if you dissociate to a degree that no longer feels healthy or safe. I did this when I got up and went to the bathroom to cry. Although it might not feel true, you have the right to make choices about your body at all times.

Third, when you are in a yoga class, you, and you alone, get to decide whether it's okay for a teacher to touch or adjust you in your poses. Don't worry about hurting their feelings. If they are mindful at what they do, they'll understand that you're taking care of yourself. They have other ways to assist you, including verbal cueing.

And finally, make sure you have support, be patient and loving with yourself as you explore the stories that live within your body, and know that getting triggered on the mat is a very normal part of the process. However, being re-traumatized and remaining in overwhelm is neither healthy nor useful. So, again, know that you can come out of the pose, get off your mat, leave the room, take a walk, or grab a friend to stay with you—no shame, no blame. You have agency, and you get to decide.

It's really not that unusual for emotions to run amok like mine did, trying to find a place to land and something to justify their uprising when tension is released—and it certainly happens as much off the mat as on. But here's the thing: even when our minds wander off on a tangent and we haven't a clue what's causing the shitstorm brewing inside, the body continues to alert us through physiological cues, which we can easily misinterpret. I know I'm hardly the only one who has felt irritated toward someone or something, not because they deserved it, but because something else was irritating or pissing me off that I couldn't identify or wasn't even aware of. So often feelings like these are simply harbingers of something deeper trapped inside, desperate to get our attention—but we can misinterpret the signals and project our feelings elsewhere. That is what I did to "LA Girl," the young woman I judged, who was on the mat next to mine.

But why would being in a yoga pose that long cause all these feelings to surface in the first place? Why would releasing the tension I felt in my hip liberate deeply held emotions I wasn't even aware I had? Because it's the tension in the muscles, and restrictions in the connective tissue that have sealed off emotions we can't deal with, feelings that we deem "negative" or "inappropriate" or too hot to handle. Once the tension is released, the emotions rush to the surface ready to be acknowledged, dealt with, and set free.

Of course all muscular tension isn't caused by emotional stuckness or laden with unprocessed crap from your childhood. Sometimes the tension is structural, habitual, or even situational (the result of an injury, perhaps). Sometimes emotions arise, sometimes they don't; sometimes muscles are simply tight and need to loosen up. Yoga simply says pay attention to what's happening, as it's happening, and notice your reaction to it. Your reactivity is key. There's a saying, "If it's hysterical, it's historical," which means the release of tension can elicit strong reactions that have nothing to do with what's going on in the moment; rather, they are rooted in childhood or even ancestral traumas.

In the same way you inherit the color of your eyes, a taste for spicy food, or the texture of your hair, you inherit the experiences, traditions, beliefs, and traumas of the people who came before you. The suppressed energy, unresolved, lived within them, affecting their health, wellness, and perspective, especially if they experienced chronic stress or feared for their survival. As that energy lived within them, so it lives within you as well. We are all directly, although often unconsciously, influenced by our ancestors' repressed stressors and beliefs, which shape the way we experience ourselves and the world around us.

Sometimes you might have an emotional reaction or release in your practice, which is fine; sometimes you don't, which is also fine. There's really no blueprint, no place to get to, and nobody's experience is any better, worse, or less authentic than anyone else's. The focus is on the moment-to-moment experiences, not the endpoint. And seriously? The last thing I want to imply is that every time you take a yoga class, you'll have a big emotional catharsis and wind up bolting from the room in tears!

What all muscular tension does do, however, is restrict the flow of energy and cause either physical or emotional discomfort—or both. Any sensation you experience—a sharp pain in the hip, tightness in the jaw, a racing heartbeat, constriction in the throat—can alert you to emotions buried within the tension. Sensations aren't the emotions themselves; rather, they're the body's way of communicating with you, getting your attention, letting you know something's bubbling up that you should investigate: *Is it harmful? Is it pleasurable? Is it troubling? Is this physical? Is this something else that needs to be explored?* A tight jaw might mean anger; a racing heart could communicate fear; constriction in the throat could signal sadness or even rage; pain in the hip could indicate an old injury or a need to shift position. The mind tries to assign meaning to these sensations, labeling them either positive or negative. If they're more than we can handle, it will revert to its favorite distraction techniques to avoid discomfort. Off the mat, that might mean food, sex, drugs, alcohol, shopping, or binging on TV or the Internet. On the mat, we might engage in fantasy, fidget, create to-do lists, judge, or compare ourselves to someone else, or think about food, alcohol, drugs, or sex.

The body, however, isn't the least bit interested in unpacking the narrative, or labeling sensations as "positive" or "negative" or even "past," "present," or "future." Sensations are neutral, nothing more than energy; in fact, the word *emotions* comes from the Latin word *emotere*, which means "to move out of." The body's job is to keep the energy moving and the channels clear. All it wants to do is to find or create safety in the moment; it is not interested in, or even capable of, processing or making sense of anything.

When energy is moving, we feel spacious, expansive, and free. Feelings arise, they abide, and they dissolve. When we experience feelings we can't handle—feelings we're ashamed of or that are layered with meaning from old traumas and past experiences we haven't dealt with—we feel narrow, contracted, and stressed. Energy builds up, and we don't know how to get it moving again. The first place affected is the nervous system. When we experience something that overwhelms us, we go into fight-flight-freeze-fold mode—which is perfectly natural. But

if we are unable or unwilling to deal with the overwhelming experience—by raging, crying, shaking, yawning, or otherwise discharging the energy—the feelings move into the muscles, which constrict around the pain in the form of muscular tension. If we continue to repress the emotions, that tension increases and moves into the connective tissues (the fascia) and the organs. The fascia—basically the shrink-wrap of the body that holds everything together—becomes congested, thick, and stiff from the burden of holding the pain of those memories and the scars from our past experiences and those of our ancestors, all of which further restrict the flow of energy. Unlike muscles, connective tissue should never be stretched through repetitive action. It takes stillness and time to regain elasticity, long holds to effect change.

Unfortunately, by the time our emotions get lodged in the connective tissue, they are much more difficult to identify and discharge. We might think we're enraged, but if we can stay with the sensations bubbling up, we may discover that the rage, a more familiar and often safer emotion, is actually masking fear, or perhaps even grief.

RELEASING TENSION

The way to get energy moving again is to release tension in the muscles, to untie the knots in the fascia that keep your emotions on lock-down. Asana definitely helps you do that, but only when you honor your physiological and emotional limitations, never going beyond what the body can handle. That's called *playing the edge*, and it's an important concept to remember. The edge is that place in a pose between intensity and pain. Physical pain—a sharp, electric sensation that causes the body to recoil and the breath to shorten—is never okay. Emotional overwhelm— feelings like panic or extreme agitation—is never okay. Intensity, on the other hand, invites expansion, curiosity, a let's-stay-here-and-explore attitude; there's room for the breath to deepen and slow down. The initial edge of a pose is where your body naturally stops when it begins to feel the stretch. Stay there, feel, breathe, and listen. And then, play a little. Can you go a bit deeper? How does *that* feel? Relax any muscular effort and simply breathe there. The intensity is fine as long as you can breathe smoothly and evenly and—most important—as long as

you feel safe. Your maximum edge is just *before* the stretch turns into pain and you begin to contract; before "ahh, that feels good" or "ohh, that feels intense" becomes "shit, that hurts!"

You must pay attention to your physical alignment too. Not because you have to rock a picture-perfect pose, but because you must counter the body's natural tendency to bend where it is soft and ignore places where it feels stiff and constricted. Without proper alignment, you can fall into habitual patterns that exploit mobility and increase rigidity—at the same time. When that happens, you not only run the risk of physical injury, but you make it more difficult to access those contracted places where the emotions reside. The fact is, you need to find a way into those "forbidden" areas. You need to create tension—exert muscular effort, in other words—in order to release tension, increase blood flow, and liberate the emotions buried there. Proper alignment helps by providing more structural stability, and mindful awareness helps by engaging with whatever arises—without judgment.

Like many people, I grew up being afraid of my big emotions. As a sensitive child, I responded differently to the world than my brothers did. I was a big feeler and needed space to be with and understand my emotions, but I wasn't given the tools to do that. Instead, I was often shamed and unintentionally instructed not to trust my instincts. So, I suppressed those big emotions and depended on the tension of that suppression to keep control of my body. By the time I was a young adult, the big feelings didn't really align with the image I wanted the world to see, anyway. Whenever they'd surface, I'd just push them back down. They were too messy and certainly not in keeping with my yogic self. I was spiritual, damn it. I wanted people to see that I was compassionate, altruistic, loving, and "living in the light", in order for that to happen, I needed to control my narrative. There was no place in that storyline for my shame or my rage or the behaviors I wasn't proud of—like the way I was critical and often judged others, or myself, as weak or ridiculous or bothersome. These emotions clouded the light; they were part of what is called the "shadow self," and I worked hard to deny them an opportunity to emerge. My self-image, my ego, depended upon that.

STANDING IN THE SHADOW

We all have a shadow self—qualities within our personality we believe are bad, wrong, or naughty. These can include greed, perversion, shame, rage, guilt—even jealousy, impatience, anger, and sexual feelings, depending on the explicit and implicit lessons we learned in childhood. In spite of our best efforts to keep these parts of ourselves hidden away, they reveal themselves in both subtle and overt ways when we are off our center. When they do surface, we may feel even worse about ourselves, believing we're the only ones who have ever acted or felt this way and are obviously majorly screwed up.

But guess what? Our shadow is a fundamental part of our humanity, absolutely essential for our evolution and growth. To deny it diminishes our capacity to embrace the power of our light. Shadow work can give us a glimpse into our ego, allowing us to transcend these aspects with awareness and compassion. Many things determine the depths of our attachment and relationship to our shadow self, including trauma, upbringing, cultural conditioning, religious fundamentalism, PTSD, or other psychological imbalances. To be clear, though, if we have an ego—and we all do—then we also have a shadow self. Our work is to understand our shadow, be in relationship to it, and work with it to move toward self-understanding, reconciliation, and healing. Our shadow has a great many things to teach us.

Our shadow helps us to remember that everything is energy; everything has a vibration; and everything needs space to move, shift, and release. Cyndi Dale, energy healer and author of *The Subtle Body*, defines energy as "vibration with information." This book is energy; so is a computer or a cup of tea—these are examples of energy you can see and interact with. And, there are forms of energy you can't see, but you definitely experience them: energies like thoughts and feelings, including love and joy, as well as fear, rage, and grief. All energies have an effect on our bodies and our minds.

Repressed emotions are energy that has no space to move, shift, and release. When something triggers them, they either burst forth or burrow further down. If they do explode, the release can feel good, at least

temporarily. But we must face them when they surface, otherwise their newly released energy can make us critical, judgmental, confrontational, aggressive, or even withdrawn or shut down. This behavior is an impulsive (or shadow) reaction to the shadow emotions begging to be heard, which creates more fear, more hate—and more separation. The opposite of yoga. Unless we process these deeper emotions, they stay within us and impact our life and our health, or they get projected outward, affecting our relationships and our work in the world. You can't run from what is within you. The shadow self is not bad; all it's asking is to be understood.

My shadow self was running the show that day in Bryan's class. My shadow reaction to the emotions bubbling up inside of me was to project them all onto the woman practicing next to me, which kept me from investigating my own internalized trauma. In my head I criticized, judged, and ridiculed her and felt totally justified. If only her behavior would change, then I would feel better. Of course, the anger I felt had absolutely nothing to do with her, but when you're triggered, when you're in your shadow, it's almost impossible to recognize that. All you know is you're annoyed, and it must be someone else's fault.

This push-me, pull-me tug-of-war with our good-self, bad-self image happens when we are "stuck in our ego," as Bryan used to say. But what does that even mean? We are told to "transcend" the ego, stop identifying with it, but how do we do that when we're not really sure what it is we're identifying with or turning away from?

WORKING WITH THE EGO

You have an ego for a reason. It's your self-image, your personality, the identity you take on. It would be next to impossible to live without one; the ego helps you navigate the world and be a friend, a parent, a lover, a productive human being. The ego is called *ahamkara* in Sanskrit, which means "I-ness" or the "I-maker." It's the identification you have with the physical body, other people, and the world around you through your five senses and your mind. The ego includes your judgments, projections, prejudices, biases, labels, titles, roles, and even

the masks you wear to hide your true self—and your shadow self.

Having an ego isn't a problem—in fact, to deny the ego is to deny our own humanity. But over-identifying with it is, believing our own hype is, and separating ourselves from (or pitting ourselves against) others is. B.K.S. Iyengar calls this "falling for the impersonation of our Soul by our ego." When we are in our ego, we become obsessed with our narrative, one we carefully curate and manage. There is no room for the shadow. We love a good, self-aggrandizing storyline—like *I'm the strongest and most flexible practitioner in this studio*, or *I'm a loving mom (dad, friend, partner)*—and, outwardly at least, we identify with it 100 percent. Our self-worth and self-confidence depend on it being true. But that can backfire.

Let me ask you this: What if you aren't what you project? If you define yourself as a loving partner, for example, what happens when you have one of those days when you're not so "loving," when you feel like a raging bitch or an arrogant asshole? Who are you then? A failure? If you pin your worth on external or material things—the amount of money you have, the relationship you're in, what you're capable of doing—when any of that collapses, your self-worth collapses along with it. When you feel ashamed, less-than, or a failure, do you ever feel unworthy of your own love—or other people's? When you become too self-absorbed, as I discovered, it's impossible to separate who you are (your true nature, your higher Self) from the limitations of your narrative (your ego, your small self).

From a spiritual perspective, getting stuck in the ego's clutches means that we consider ourselves to be somehow unique, which keeps us separate from others and from God. Of course, yoga teaches that everything is connected and that this "separation" we perceive is, in fact, an illusion. But we can't move into these higher states of consciousness without first understanding the ego, anticipating it, and working with it. After all, we can't change what we won't see.

You can begin to work with the ego by practicing what yogis call witness consciousness—noticing what is happening without judging it, dissociating from it, or assigning meaning to it. Simply being present and listening to what comes up. The problem with all of this witnessing and listening is that the body's cues are muted and nuanced, making them difficult to decipher, so you'll need to dive deeper than simply "performing" postures. Asana is important, of course: it provides the container for self-reflection, and it can show you where the tension lies, where muscles feel tight and resistant. Pranayama then allows you to breathe your attention into the places that are knotted with anxiety and pain and to soften the sensations that arise. That's what I did in Bryan's class after I emerged from the bathroom. I became so absorbed in my experience that everything else fell away—nothing on the outside could distract me. Instead of breathing just long enough for my anxiety and "patterning" to lessen so I could function, I got quiet. I committed to watching and waiting for whatever wanted to surface. At one point, I ceased being in control; I stopped consciously placing my attention or directing my breath to specific places. I simply allowed the breath to breathe me open, to unlock, unwind, and unburden.

CONNECTING THE MIND AND THE BODY

So how can you shut out all the distractions and come to such a place of deep inquiry? By practicing pratyahara, the fifth of the eight limbs of yoga. Of course, I had no idea that day in Bryan's class that that's what I was doing; all I knew was I didn't want to interrupt the process. I was ready to listen without making any judgments and without worrying about what else was going on around me.

Pratyahara is what connects the outer and inner aspects of yoga and helps us make sense of our experiences. We can't expect a daily asana practice to help liberate us from our traumas and our suffering. That's too big of a leap. We need to develop the mind-body connection first, and we do that, according to yoga scholar David Frawley, by gaining mastery over the breath and the senses, which are what link the mind and the body in the first place. An asana practice definitely releases muscular tension, but without engaging the mind and without paying attention to it all, letting go of that tension could be scary. It could allow sensations to arise that we're not prepared to feel or deal with. As a young adult, I often found contracting around sensation useful; the tension in my muscles helped me contain the energy so I could take things slow and remain safe and more in control. But, by the time I left the bathroom during Bryan's class that day, I was ready for the deeper wisdom my emotional release would reveal.

Witness consciousness comes from your heart center, awakens your intuition, and puts your judgments, fears, and insecurities on hold. It is where you can practice equanimity, that sense of calm abiding Bryan talked about in class. Some Buddhists translate equanimity as both "seeing with patience" and "standing in the middle." Bryan invited his class to be equanimous—present to what comes up without shutting down, reacting, or resisting. He encouraged us to stay in witness consciousness, to connect to our own true essence, which is God, basic goodness, or Universal Consciousness—to see the beauty in all that we are.

I made a commitment that day to listen and to focus on the sensations themselves, to notice where these sensations lived in my body, acknowledge them, and let them release.

As those stuck places inside me began to open up, images and colors emerged, memories arose, and my body began to speak: it needed to tell its story; it needed me to give voice to all parts of me, including the beautiful little girl I had once been. We cannot ignore the story, we cannot transcend it, until we are in relationship to it. To invite those places to surface is the only way we can heal the separation within ourselves, liberate ourselves from our ego, and allow the soul to evolve. It's not easy—it takes patience and compassion and a belief that there is a place for everything within you. But the cool thing about yoga is you don't have to do it all at once. You can stop whenever you want to and start again when it feels safe. It's truly about bringing the mind, the body, and the heart together to bear witness to all that you are—with love.

THE GONG OF AWAKENING

6

ONE MORNING WHEN I was working behind the desk at the studio, a woman came in I had never seen before. She was beautiful, maybe around fifty, dressed all in white, and wearing a turban with a large topaz pinned at the center. She signed her name, looked up at me, and smiled. She introduced herself as Gurmukh Kaur Khalsa and asked me my name. Something about her intrigued me, so I decided to take the same class she was taking. I rolled out my mat far enough from hers so she wouldn't think I was stalking her—but close enough to see her. I watched as she removed her turban, allowing her long hair to fall all around her. In one quick move, she casually swept it up in a bun and secured it with a white kerchief. She then removed her tunic to reveal leggings and a form-fitting bodysuit underneath—white, of course. She looked over at me and smiled. I smiled back and quickly looked away, feeling a tad creepy for staring at her. I immediately liked this woman, although I had no idea why. She stepped onto her mat and joined the rest of us as the teacher lead the class through some down and dirty hardcore flow. She was a remarkable practitioner, elegant and strong.

99

During the meditation at the end of class, I snuck a peek and saw her effortlessly disappear into some other world. Her eyes rolled up and back, and she was completely immersed in her own experience with the Divine—at least that's what it looked like to me. When I asked a few friends about her, I learned that Gurmukh, who hailed from a small town in Illinois, was arguably the most powerful teacher of Kundalini yoga in the States. She had become a Sikh after meeting Yogi Bhajan, an entrepreneur and master of Kundalini yoga, who arrived in the United States from India in the late '60s.

I went home and read all I could find about Kundalini yoga and about Yogi Bhajan. He often wrote about the chakras—or energy centers in the body—as a pathway to Spirit and the states of ecstasy you can achieve when you've cleared the blockages. I decided I wanted to learn more, so I drove to Golden Bridge Yoga, in the center of Los Angeles, to take a class with Gurmukh.

▼

Golden Bridge is a beautiful school, open and airy, and just like my experience at Integral Yoga in New York City, most everyone there (except me) is dressed all in white. Some have yoga mats spread out on the floor, with a small cushion called a *zafu* perched toward the top end. Others rest on thick white sheepskin carpets, which, as an animal lover, is not my favorite thing to see. A massive gong hangs from the wall near the front of the room; I wonder how they plan to use that thing in our asana class. Figuring it'll be loud and distracting, I move my mat as far away from it as possible.

Gurmukh enters the room from somewhere on high, wearing a loose, white gown, with sheer pale gold panels of chiffon draped around her shoulders. She looks like an angel, and I'm pretty sure she just floated across the room. She has a regal air about her, and yet she pauses to say hello, to kiss, and to touch hands with everyone she passes as she makes her way to the stage. She spots me, smiles, leans down to kiss my cheek, telling me how pleased she is to see me again, and gently strokes my hair.

She remembers me! I kinda fall in love with her right then and there.

Until we begin practicing the *kriyas*.

Kriyas are various postures, pranayama, mantra, and vocalization techniques used to stimulate the subtle energy bodies. These repetitive movements, almost always practiced with an experienced teacher, can induce what yogis call a Kundalini rising, which helps the student reach climatic states of awareness—or so I'd been told. I hadn't been told, however, that they'd require so much endurance. I just figured we'd be throwing down some sun salutes and a bunch of standing poses, like in every other class I go to. Nope. Not at all.

Instead, Gurmukh, sitting crossed-legged and serene, asks us to hold our arms up over our heads in a *V* shape, our hands in a fist and our thumbs pointed upward, for what seems like fifteen minutes straight—in other words, forever. In the meantime, with the music blasting the chant "Wahe Guru" over and over again, she calls out prompts to keep us motivated, encouraging us to chant along, the tempo getting increasingly faster. The music finally dies down, so I figure we'll get a little relief, but instead she instructs us to bend the elbows and clasp the hands behind the neck. The music cranks up again, and we twist our torsos from side to side while panting hard through the mouth—for *another* fifteen minutes. A bunch more stuff equally and unbearably hard follows, which drains the blood from my appendages and leaves me dizzy.

Gurmukh leads us through all this so effortlessly, as if it's the most natural thing in the world, her chiffon panels floating in rhythm, a sweet smile on her face. Me, on the other hand? I am pouring sweat and can't believe no one warned me about this. Kundalini is freaking hard. Even with all my strength from Power Yoga, just keeping my arms up is impossibly difficult. I look around the room to see if anyone else is struggling and am happy to see that they are! What a relief to know that I'm not out of shape or that my mind isn't making this harder than it's supposed to be. Fact: it is *really* hard!

After about an hour, moving and breathing in a specific way, chanting mantra and various sounds, my body is buzzing, and I am exhausted. Gurmukh stands up and glides across the floor toward the gong. *Oh God, not the gong.* She asks us to sit tall and close our eyes. My body's still pulsating; I feel twitchy, and the tips of my fingers and toes have gone numb. I shake out my hands before resting them on my knees, my palms facing up.

Gurmukh tells us to assume the *gyan mudra*, which means we place our thumb and index finger together, with the other fingers extending straight out.

She invites us to close our eyes and bring our attention to the base of the spine, to the *muladhara* chakra, directly at the perineum. She asks us to feel into our roots and into the earth beneath us, into the connection we have to each other and to the planet. "Notice," she says, "what might be blocking you from uniting in love with your family, your tribe, this planet, and one another." She explains that a strong foundation is critical to our health and to our spiritual upliftment. I bring my attention downward.

Lifting the cloth-covered stick she's holding in her hand, Gurmukh gently hits the gong. The tone is deep and low and reverberates through the room. The vibration strikes me deep in my legs and pelvis, like a weight pulling me downward, and I let it. With my attention concentrated in the lowest part of my spine, I easily see the color red when she invites us to visualize it.

I suddenly imagine a thick red cord that moves from deep within my spine into the earth beneath me, anchoring me to the floor, allowing my spine to lift higher and the top of my head to extend off of my neck. My body continues to respond to the crescendo of the gong's vibration.

After a while, the sound softens a bit, and Gurmukh directs our attention to the lower part of the abdomen, in front of the sacrum, and asks us to bring forth the color orange. This, she explains, is the second chakra, *svadhisthana*, our creative center, where we embody our sexuality and our emotions, where we give birth, both literally and figuratively. She hits the gong again.

The sound of the gong spreads through my pelvis, genitals, and hips, entering into my muscles, bones, and connective tissues, making everything come alive, pleasurable, expansive, deep, and ancient. I feel a swirl of energy, fluid and feminine—which makes sense as soon as I hear her say that this chakra is associated with the water element. I move deeper into the sound of the gong and listen for Gurmukh's instructions.

"Notice what arises," I hear her say through the deep resonance of the gong. Or gongs? Were there other gongs in the room that I didn't see? The sound seems to be hitting me from all sides.

"Bring your awareness to the *manipura* chakra, your self-esteem, your ego, your power center. See the color yellow," she says as she strikes the gong. The pitch seems higher and lands right at my center. The heat within me increases; I feel drunk with pleasure and begin to giggle. The color yellow fills the whole of my awareness.

"Focus your attention to your heart center, to the *anahata* chakra! The element is air. See the color green. This is our center of love. Of forgiveness. Of empathy and compassion. Let it fill you!" The gong rings out loudly.

I raise my awareness to my heart center, and I feel it expand across my chest. My body jerks slightly, but I continue breathing through it, each inhale drawing energy from my base up higher through my spine, each exhale grounding me, the energy cord connecting my body with the earth beneath. I feel so utterly present *and* out of my fucking mind.

Gurmukh calls out for us to place our attention on the *vishuddha* chakra, the throat center. My breath moves up higher, my neck and jaw lifting off my shoulders. But instead of feeling expansive, I feel my energy contract; it's stuck and locked up. I breathe in deeply, open my mouth wide and take a lion's breath, extending my tongue out and making a sound. I figure no one can hear me over the gong anyway. The release of energy from my mouth and jaw brings tears to my eyes. It feels so good to let the energy out, so necessary. So I take another one, then another, until the energy finally breaks free and moves up my cervical spine.

It's now time to lift our eyeballs up to the third eye, the *ajna* chakra. This is the point of intuition, Gurmukh tells us, the place where we are guided from within, the repository of all our visions, dreams, and prophetic thoughts. As the gong's pitch changes once again, I turn my eyes upward. I feel a jolt of energy rip from the base of my spine and land at the center point of my brows. Holy shit. The energy is so intense, so pleasurable, that I wonder if I'm having an orgasm. But the sensation is not centered in my genitals—it's expanding right at my heart center. Everything within me and around me begins to dissolve. I feel as though I'm falling into the sound of the gong. My head begins to sway back and forth on my neck, and I'm pretty sure I'm about to tip over onto the floor.

The gong's tone changes again. I hear Gurmukh's voice from far away telling us to focus on the crown of the head, the seventh and final chakra, the *sahasrara* chakra. I do. A bright, golden light fills my entire body, which shakes and jerks forward. That orgasmic feeling bursts through me again, and I am wrapped in pure pleasure, joy, and beauty. I have no desire to analyze or try to make sense of any of it; I simply let the sound and the emotions envelop me. All I know is that I am bliss; I am infinite.

The sounds of the gong begin to fade, and we are left in silence. I am sure my mouth is gaping open. I might even be drooling. I don't know and don't care. I am overcome with a feeling of connection. I never want this to end.

Gurmukh tells us to sit with what we feel.

I feel everything. I feel nothing. I am hovering in the space between each breath.

From somewhere in the room I hear singing.

> May the longtime sun shine upon you,
> All love surround you,
> And the pure light within you,
> Guide your way on . . .

Tears are streaming down my face, but I am smiling, my mouth stretched tightly across my face. It must be the biggest smile any face has ever smiled.

I hear Gurmukh once again ask what we feel.

God. I feel God.

TEACHINGS FROM THE ZAFU
THE SUBTLE BODY, CHAKRAS, AND METAPHYSICS

So much happened in Gurmukh's class. Where do I even begin? It was definitely a moment of initiation, during which I not only felt the power of all the chakras for the first time, but I also had my first Kundalini awakening. All kinds of things can happen during such an awakening. You may experience a surge of energy that electrifies the whole body and causes jerking, twitching, shaking, or heat rising; a feeling that you are one with everything and everyone; an expansion of the heart so it holds more compassion than you ever thought possible. When all that's going on, yogis say, the subtle energy body (the pranamaya kosha I talked about earlier) is being stimulated, and the prana is charging up through the chakra system, opening all the channels and giving us a glimpse into transcendent states of awareness. And yes, it's as cool as it sounds. The profound release of stagnant energy shifts our consciousness from density into liberation, uniting matter and consciousness as one. It is wondrous!

All those kriyas Gurmukh taught—especially the ones where I thought my arms would fall off—activate the chakras, the energy centers in the body. By the time I took my seat for meditation, my awareness had expanded into places I never knew existed. My sense of ego, of I-ness, fell away, and I felt a profound sense of connection within me and with everything around me. A new sense of spaciousness created a shift in my subtle energy body, which seemed to be having quite the time of it. Colors, images, and flashes of light rushed in as energy rose up from the base of my spine to the crown of my head. I felt whole. I felt God. I felt love with every fiber of my being. And I never wanted to be separated from my true nature again.

You release the ego, the shadow self, through self-reflection, self-acceptance, and forgiveness. When you forgive someone, you release the caustic energy of resentment and the prana can begin to flow steadily through the *nadis* (energy pathways) and the chakras (psychic energy centers). You can untangle unconscious patterns and behaviors, bathe your cells and auric field (the energy field that surrounds the body) with life-force, and awaken to Universal Consciousness and your true potential. Forgiveness is absolutely fundamental to your spiritual growth and to your freedom, as I discovered again and again, but I had only gotten a taste of its power to heal. Just because I was able to forgive myself in Bryan's class doesn't mean I was done or that I had issued a blanket forgiveness statement that would carry me through everything I had yet to face. Forgiveness is a process, a lifelong endeavor.

What also happened in Gurmukh's class was that I suddenly found myself understanding ancient concepts viscerally, concepts that I had struggled to grasp. These truths revealed themselves from deep within. They showed me that when I release the tension, reconcile the limiting beliefs and stories I am carrying, I can free the channels of energy and begin to "hear" not from my head and ego, but from my heart and actualized Self.

Although all this talk about nadis and chakras sounds so esoteric, so magical, it really isn't. It's yoga's way of describing the consequences of our felt experiences. As I have already shared, everything

you do, everything you think, feel, and remember—your joys, sorrows, longings, traumas—all of it impacts your physical body, your thoughts, and your emotions. But, as I discovered, it goes beyond the physical-mental realm (the body and the thinking mind) and hits you up on a psycho-spiritual level (the intuitive mind and spirit) in the subtle energy body as well. There, it either allows for the free flow of vital energy within and among the chakras, or it sets up roadblocks and detours that prevent you from realizing true spiritual connection.

When you get triggered, when you're in your shit and can't get out of it, you already know what happens in the physical-mental realm: your reactions affect the autonomic nervous system, and you get stuck in fight-flight-freeze-fold (the sympathetic response, or SNS). A similar thing happens in the subtle energy body. Although the pranamaya kosha has thousands of nadis, there are three main ones: *ida*, *pingala*, and *sushumna*. The ida nadi loosely corresponds to the parasympathetic, or rest-and-digest response (PNS). A balanced ida nadi makes you feel calm, centered, and connected to your feelings. When this pathway gets blocked by stress, fear, anxiety, and other strong emotions, it brings on feelings of being disconnected, depressed, suspicious, and weepy. A balanced pingala nadi, which loosely corresponds to the SNS, ensures that you are awake, active, and energized; when it's blocked, you can easily become agitated or moody, quick to judge and blame.

Just like the PNS and the SNS, the ida and pingala dominate at different times, reacting and responding to everything that's going on around and within you, and just like their physiological counterparts, they can easily be destabilized.

The sushumna nadi is the flow of energy, centered deep within the spinal column, that begins at the base of the spine and moves upward, connecting the seven energy centers, from the root chakra to the crown chakra. Unlike the ida and pingala, the sushumna is immune to the force field of energies surrounding it. Its energy is pure, joyful, and unadulterated. However, in order for the energy to move freely up the sushumna, the ida and the pingala— the subtle energy body's nervous system—must be balanced.

Chakras, fusions of electromagnetic energy, result whenever the ida and pingala intersect along the sushumna pathway. These chakras connect the physical-mental body with the psycho-spiritual body. Although none of this is visible or detectable, make no mistake: the effects the nadis and chakras have on your well-being are profound. Your immune system, nervous system, organ function, emotions, and spiritual development all depend on these energy centers being open and balanced.

Each chakra has its own energy frequency, color, and sound and is responsible for specific physiological functions. Each chakra also absorbs the psychic and emotional residue of every moment, each experience, and all beings who affect our lives. Our own narratives and those of our families, culture, gender, sexuality, and religion, along with any accumulated trauma, both personal and ancestral, directly influence the vibrational quality of each chakra and determine the rate at which it spins (excessive, deficient, or balanced). If that residue cannot be processed and discharged, it will prevent prana from flowing optimally through the chakra, adversely affecting it and all the other chakras as well. When the chakras are affected, the body is affected too. When the body is affected, so is the mind. And when the mind is affected, it is impossible to get out of our own way to "listen" to the internal messages we receive.

Bringing the subtle energy body back into balance requires asana and pranayama practices that target specific areas of the body. That makes perfect sense because each chakra directly affects specific parts of our anatomy by bringing prana or life force there. It's pretty obvious that controlling and extending the breath—increasing vital energy—has a profound impact on the subtle energy body. But what about asana? How does asana help?

Remember that everything you feel, including the shadow emotions you have trouble acknowledging, lives in the body, and if you don't allow your feelings to arise and then dissolve, they will become stuck there, taking up residence in places like the hips, the jaw, the shoulders. By creating distinct shapes through asana, you can move your awareness and your breath into those areas and encourage the energy to release. All of this helps you understand what your body is trying to tell you and offers you clues on how to bring these embodied "stories" into your awareness, and hopefully assist in your own healing.

However, it's not enough to do the poses and discharge energy. You need to go back to witness consciousness and investigate how these blockages got there in the first place. What story is hiding underneath the tension? What is it trying to teach you? Only when you enter into a relationship with your stories, with your discomfort, can you release the suppressed emotions safely.

When I was in Bryan's class, I experienced an emotional catharsis in Pigeon Pose, a common hip opener. Looking back, I shouldn't have been surprised. So many of my suppressed emotions, my trauma, and my self-image, which centered around sexual molestation and betrayal, live in the lower part of the body—the hips, the pelvis, the intestinal tract, and the legs. The discomfort I felt was more than just physical; it was emotional; it was primal. The images arising from my past and the colors I saw were all centered around home, safety, survival, fear, and physicality—concerns related to the first chakra. The tension emanating from my hips stemmed from betrayal, sex, abuse, abandonment, and guilt, and kept me separate and distrustful of the world around me—second chakra stuff. As I began to allow the energy to rise up and out of me, I vowed to stay present and fully feel everything. The insights I received while in the pose were directly in alignment with the bottom two chakras. There was a direct connection between what I was "seeing" and the part of my body that was releasing. As I can attest, the chakra system can help you make emotional connections, provides insight, and allows you to work through blockages with both physical structure and symbolic guidance.

THE CHAKRAS AND OUR TRAUMA

The chakras don't only hold on to all the messy stuff, they also contain the residue from everything wondrous and positive in our lives. Unfortunately, the good stuff gets harder to access when our shadow emotions block the way. Understanding the psychic damage that trauma inflicts on the chakras can help us direct prana into those areas that need to be liberated in order for us to be whole.

Of course, what follows is hardly a deep dive into the chakras—that would be an entire book in itself. Instead, I'm focusing on the relationship between the chakras and personal and ancestral trauma in hopes that it will give you some insight about your own journey and how you can explore these centers on the yoga mat. I'll share a bit about each chakra, including the various narratives that can affect it, the shadow emotions that are associated with it, and the body parts it influences. I'll then focus on what happens when it becomes destabilized. Having said that, the best way to understand the chakras is by experiencing them, so get on your mat and practice!

Muladhara Chakra (The Root)

Located at the base of your spine (or the perineum), the root chakra helps you remain grounded and secure in the physical world—home, safety, and stability—and governs your survival instinct as you navigate your place in society and on the planet. It is what roots us to each other and to the here and now. It exhibits a primal force, teaching you how to be in your body, how to live in relationship—and sustain it—with the world, your family, and your tribe. Not surprisingly, this is where much of your trauma is initiated, including developmental and ancestral traumas. Trauma is the earthquake that shakes our foundation, ripping the ground right out from under us. Although the magnitude of this internal quake is particularly acute when the abuse or other trauma happens in childhood—when our world revolves around those who are supposed to care for and protect us—all unresolved trauma disrupts this chakra. And, sadly, a crack in the foundation makes the entire structure unsound. If the first chakra is blocked, all the rest are too, since our foundation is responsible for supporting the whole of our being.

Shadow: Fear

Location: Legs, feet, rectum, spinal column, lower intestinal tract, bones, teeth, and immune system

Personal Traumas: Pregnancy or birth trauma, abandonment, ableism, rejection, lack of proper nourishment, incarceration, being in threatening environments or witnessing violence (including physical abuse), homelessness

Inherited Traumas: Family members who were survivors of genocide or colonization; enslaved people and enslavers, or war veterans; domestic violence, those who experienced gang violence, racism, segregation, displacement, or forced immigration and poverty

Svadhisthana Chakra (The Sacral)

Located below the navel, this chakra governs how you relate to yourself and how you relate to others. It determines how you experience and honor your sexuality and your creativity, whether you're making babies or making your mark in the world. It's pretty easy to see how trauma's vibrational energy can compromise this one. When you don't have a loving relationship with yourself, when you don't trust that you are worthy of love from others, you may not be able to create healthy boundaries; you may consistently put yourself in harm's way by choosing abusive partners or ones who aren't emotionally available, or you may compromise yourself in exchange for sex, drugs, money, power, or influence. These are all the ways in which we give ourselves away because we lack the support and stability we need to be fully awake and present, independent of a relationship with someone else.

Shadow: Guilt

Location: Sexual organs, hips and pelvic area, intestines, and bladder

Personal Traumas: Sexual, emotional, or physical abuse; ageism; emotional exploitation; abortion or miscarriage; religious zealotry or moral rigidity; having a parent or parents with a substance-use disorder

Inherited Traumas: Parents or ancestors who have suppressed or haven't dealt with their own sexual issues; those who were punished because of their sexual or gender identity or behavior; other trauma related to their sexuality or gender, such as sex trafficking or cults, rape, prostitution, homophobia, transphobia, misogyny, sexism, and abuse

Manipura Chakra (The Solar Plexus)

Located in the solar plexus, this energy center is where you begin to individuate from the collective and develop your personal power, your sense of self, independent from your tribe. Your self-confidence manifests in this vortex, and so does your ego and its attachments to the physical world, as it craves self-definition and value. When you lack confidence or get stuck in your ego, you can develop low self-worth or poor self-discipline, feel easily victimized, and be inclined to blame others and shame yourself. Low self-esteem can

also move you in the opposite direction, manifesting as emotional control and manipulative, aggressive, and even violent behavior. Someone with a manipura chakra imbalance can become deceptive, volatile, stubborn, addicted to power, arrogant, demeaning, and cruel.

Shadow: Shame

Location: The muscular system, stomach, pancreas, liver, gallbladder, spleen, and intestinal tract

Personal Traumas: Being shamed or being a victim of systemic exclusion; entering into or staying in volatile, dominating, or submissive relationships; physical abuse; emotional manipulation; and dangerous, disempowering, or oppressive situations

Inherited Traumas: Parents or ancestors who themselves have experienced abuse, including military abuse, or have been oppressed or in danger

Anahata Chakra (The Heart)

Located in the center of the chest, this chakra bridges the earthly and the spiritual, allowing you to explore the depths of emotional well-being with compassion and be present to the experience of others with empathy, understanding, and forgiveness. When unprocessed emotions or trauma mess with this chakra, they may manifest as antisocial tendencies, bitterness, hypercriticism, resentment, or lack of compassion for self and others, all of which can result in loneliness, social anxiety, depression, fear of intimacy and relationships, suspicion, and even narcissism. On the other end of the spectrum, codependency, lack of boundaries, neediness, jealousy, and martyrdom can arise.

Shadow: Grief

Location: Heart, lungs, thymus gland, breasts, shoulder blades, and arms

Personal Traumas: Experiences of rejection, humiliation, abandonment; suppressed grief; break-up, loss, or death of a loved one; withheld affection; betrayal; and sexual, emotional, or physical abuse

Inherited Traumas: Includes all the unresolved issues from the lower chakras; heartbreak, betrayal, loss, resentment, unprocessed fear, guilt, shame, and grief

Vishuddha Chakra (The Throat)

Located at the center of the throat, this chakra governs communication, self-expression, choice, and creativity. When balanced, the vishuddha chakra allows your words to reflect the inspired and loving congruence of your thoughts and your heart center. You are your most authentic self when you can speak truth with clarity, compassion, and confidence. It's pretty easy to see how being subjected to harsh criticism, verbal abuse, or hyper-strict parents or being made to keep your family's worst secrets can derail all that. When that happens, it may cause you to have a lack of trust in your own voice and be fearful of speaking up or out, which makes it difficult to communicate feelings. In excess, the fifth chakra manifests as talking too much, being critical or defensive, refusing to listen, gossiping, lying, using condescending language, and having an aggressive or dominating tone of voice.

Shadow: Lies

Location: Throat, mouth, lips, teeth, tongue, and neck

Personal Traumas: Unrestrained shouting, verbal abuse, or criticism; tyrannical or repressive parents; being the one who holds the secrets and the lies in your family

Inherited Traumas: Includes all the unresolved traumas carried in the lower chakras; threats for speaking up; submissive upbringing; social conditions where silence was critical for well-being or survival

Ajna Chakra (The Third Eye)

Located between the eyebrows, the sixth chakra, or third eye center, is where you develop your thoughts and ideas and where you begin to access your intuition, visions, and dreams. When balanced, this vortex allows you to see beyond reason, to become more intuitive, to think more symbolically, and to create meaning in your life by seeing a larger spiritual framework at play. You can trust your inner knowing and follow its mystical guidance with full faith. When trauma blocks the third eye, it may manifest as insensitivity, a distrust of intuition, lack of imagination, inability to recall your dreams, dogmatic or rigid thinking, or a weak memory. The opposite end of the spectrum includes excessive daydreaming, fantastical or obsessive thinking, nightmares, hallucinations, illusions, and inability to concentrate.

Shadow: Illusion

Location: Face, eyes, ears, and central nervous system

Personal Traumas: Being in war zones or areas of gang violence; having your intuitive wisdom or psychic experiences denied or rebutted; being told you're "crazy" for seeing or believing as you do; psychological manipulation and abuse

Inherited Traumas: Includes all unresolved trauma from the lower chakras; superstition; occult abuse; and religious dogma or control

Sahasrara Chakra (The Crown)

Located at the top of the head, the seventh chakra is where you awaken to grace. When you transcend the pull of your ego and the attachments you have to the physical world, when you learn the life lessons that have kept you bound to your shadow self, you ultimately reach a state of true bliss. When you are balanced in this vital energy center, you are wise, you are open-minded, you have a sense of spiritual connection, and you can experience yourself, each other, the planet, and God as unified. When unprocessed emotions or traumas block the crown, spiritual disenchantment, judgmental thinking, or spiritual apathy may result; you may have difficulty learning and grasping information or be unable to open to other belief systems. When trauma overstimulates, you may be confused, over-intellectualize, and suffer from spiritual narcissism or addiction, religious fanaticism, psychic delusions, or emotional or somatic dissociation.

Shadow: Attachment

Location: All the systems of the body, including dermal, hormonal, and nervous systems

Personal Traumas: A home life (or education) that interferes with your spiritual curiosity; spiritual abuse; occult abuse, extreme fundamentalism, being lied to or purposely given false information; having spiritual or moral beliefs invalidated, manipulated, or rejected

Inherited Traumas: All of the ancestral trauma already mentioned

Although I had read up on the chakras after I had my meltdown in Bryan's class, there's nothing quite like an emotional release to move me from an intellectual understanding to an embodied one. As my body released long-held tension in Gurmukh's class, with my permission, I became vulnerable—my worst nightmare at the time. But by deciding to stay with it, I surrendered to the unknown, and let myself be open to whatever arose. To be honest, I had no choice. I was tired of being imprisoned by my resentments, fears, and judgments. I wanted desperately to create enough space in my heart for all that I was so that someday I could forgive myself enough to truly love myself and others, and to finally, once and for all, know God.

This is the evolution of the soul. It can bring us from matter to consciousness, from contraction to release, and prepare us to honor and to behold the God within . . . and the God within all.

A STINGING REALIZATION

AFTER THAT DAY in Gurmukh's class in early 1994, my yoga began to shift beyond the body and find its way into my heart and my spirit. I felt open and inspired in a way I never had before and the changes in my life were evident—at least to me. I had caught the first real inkling of a spiritual reality that existed beyond my literal perception—and I got a glimpse of who I could be beyond the parameters of my flesh and bone. It wasn't that I was suddenly having daily mystical experiences. Hardly. But I had an intuitive sense that there was an intelligent force greater than my mind and a vibrant essence even more expansive than my soul. I hungered for a deeper relationship with it all. I craved more access to transcendent states of consciousness and a greater awareness of spirituality, and I knew there were techniques, beyond asana, that could bring me there. I just didn't know how to find them.

When Gurmukh asked us to name what we were feeling, I blurted out "God." Well, not really an *out loud* blurt, but my answer was so immediate and so surprising that it felt like it had come from the very depths of my soul and ricocheted off the walls. I was experiencing God as Divine presence, for the first time in my life—not as an intellectual exercise, but as a felt experience. This was not the God of my youth, which I could never relate to. When I was growing up, God lived "up there," separate from me and all others—omnipresent, omniscient, impersonal, and individuated, passing judgment on all "He" surveyed. He (and God was always referred to as a He with a capital *H*) was something to fear and negotiate with—and didn't seem to have anything to do with love. But here I was in Los Angeles, of all places, where periodically I could see how everything was connected to everything else and how I was a part of something so much greater and more beautiful than my small self could even comprehend. God wasn't an anthropomorphic figure; God wasn't separate; God was energy; God was everywhere! And if this mysterious energy was accessible, I wanted to know how to get me some on a more regular basis.

I remembered how Billy had pointed to Danny and Violet and all the people on the dance floor at Heaven, telling me that God was in them, in all beings, all moments, all time, all space, and all understanding. He encouraged me to "see" beyond reason so I would know the true essence of Grace, which was love. I really wanted to. I remembered looking around and nodding my head, hearing what he was saying but not feeling any of it. Why the hell couldn't I feel it, know it, embody it as truth? Billy could. Others in the yoga classes I attended seemed to as well. I'd often see students drop into what looked like some sort of ecstatic state, in which their body would tremble, and tears of gratitude would flow freely. Why were their ecstatic experiences so beautiful, almost ethereal, while mine were (more often than not) so heavy and laden with uncomfortable emotions? I wanted to know what I had to do in order to feel that connection all the time.

When I broached the subject with my friends at YogaWorks, they all agreed I needed a guru. I needed to "surrender my will" to someone who had divine access and could show me the path to enlightenment. Seriously? Surrender my will? Hadn't I already spent thousands of dollars on therapy learning how to call my power back? Why would I want to give it away again? Their advice freaked me out—and attracted me at the same time. It may seem counterintuitive, but in truth, I kinda wanted someone to tell me exactly how to live my life. A guru, my friends suggested, would be able to see my shortcomings as well as my emotional and spiritual maturity, and guide me, beyond the limitations of my ego attachments, to know the power and beauty of the Spirit that lived within the hearts of all beings.

If I had to give a bit of my power away to achieve enlightenment, so be it. Besides, all my friends were finding their gurus and surrendering themselves to their teachings—and they seemed fine. Many were so committed to their teachers that they went to live with them at ashrams, performing acts of selfless service daily, religiously reciting the mantras they received, and even getting new names, like Durgaji Sunflower or Kalima Fireflame. To be honest, with a name like Corn, I could use a new one. If a guru could do that, then sign me up!

I wanted to understand the mysteries of life. I longed for a teacher to give myself over to, someone who would take me under their wing and show me the ways of God. I wanted to lose myself in their wisdom and bask in the ways in which they had transcended their own longings, attachments, illusions, and desires. Because clearly I had not. I searched and bowed and even kissed a foot or two, waiting to feel that eyeball-rolling, *Shaktipat*-receiving call from the Divine-with-a-capital-*D* that a teacher could transmit directly from their soul straight into my heart.

It wasn't happening.

I was told my resistance was nothing more than my inability or unwillingness to let go of my ego. Until I could do that, I would never experience enlightenment, and I would be doomed to the continued cycle of birth, death, and rebirth, and the accumulated karma that comes with that.

My friends would say that obviously I wasn't *open*, and a potential guru would be able to sense that. Apparently the teacher doesn't appear until the student is ready. That really bummed me out.

By then, I was doing Ashtanga yoga and absorbed in the culture of that practice. I would get up, drive to Chuck Miller's 6 a.m. class at YogaWorks, and breathe and sweat alongside Shiva Rea, Max Strom, Annie Carpenter, Natasha Rizopoulos, and many other students who would one day become well-respected teachers in their own right. Everyone I loved and respected, loved and respected Pattabhi Jois, the Indian yoga teacher from Mysore, India, who popularized Ashtanga yoga—"Guruji," as he was affectionately known in that community. I couldn't wait to meet him. Maybe he would be my guru, too?

Around the same time, I also got turned on to the teachings of Sri Aurobindo and the Mother. I loved his writing and the way she presented it to the physical world.

Sri Aurobindo was an Indian spiritual leader and nationalist and had been imprisoned because of his political beliefs and actions. The Mother, whose name was Mirra Alfassa, was a French occultist who worked alongside him to bring life to his messaging. "Without him, I exist not," she said. "But without me, he is unmanifest." I loved that. That seemed like a true expression of relationship, and in yogic terms, an example of Shiva-Shakti, the balance between the male and female energies. He wrote in isolation all day, eventually going into seclusion until his death, and she went out and brought his essential messages to the world, adding her own self-expression and complementary vision. His poetry, her implementation, and the utopian society they had created—where all souls lived and worked together in harmony—intrigued me. They spoke to the individual and collective nature of humans in a way that felt like a process of self-discovery, and I started to wonder if maybe they were to become my spiritual teachers.

Just to be clear, Sri Aurobindo and the Mother were dead. He had left his body in 1950, and she hers in the early '70s. Their work lives on at their well-respected ashram in Pondicherry, India, where a diverse and multicultural community called Auroville continues to work together peacefully. Maybe, I thought, some of their devotees could guide me?

I decided to make a pilgrimage to India. I longed to immerse myself in a culture that lives and breathes the practice of yoga as a part of its daily life. Yoga is everywhere in India. It's in the temples, the traffic, the sheer number of people in the streets. It's in the sights and smells; it's in animals that roam freely; it's in every blessed and broken soul. India forces you to be present and demands that you pay attention to every moment as something that is sacred, something profane, something holy, something hellacious. I understood that such a pilgrimage was a necessary step on the spiritual path upon which countless others from the West had embarked well before I did. I hoped that being there, in the birthplace of yoga, I would find my own spiritual guide. Maybe in Pondicherry? Or perhaps even Mysore, at the feet of Pattabhi Jois. I landed first in Mysore, tired from the journey but eager to immerse myself in my studies and meet the guru himself.

I fell in love with India the moment I arrived—and then despised it about an hour later, only to fall madly in love with it again by the end of the day. It went on like this for months. It felt like a country of extremes, a place that seemed to hold so many dualities. India is beautiful, exotic, rich, lush, vibrant, magical, and spiritual. It is also grotesque, brutal, impoverished, unfair, depraved, dirty, and cruel. It is my favorite country in the world. I can't stand it. I can't wait to go back. When can I leave? Yeah, it's kinda like that.

India has a way of exposing those very dualities within you. The shadow and the light. India is yoga, and the lessons I learned there, very different from the West, helped me embody the practice, and its teaching, in many essential and life-transforming ways. It took traveling to India to return home to myself.

▼

The morning after I arrive in Mysore, I tuck my well-worn yoga mat under my arm and walk to the yoga shala. I'm already sweating in the 90-degree heat and it's only 7 a.m.! My heart's beating fast with excitement as I join other students from all over the world who are waiting their turn on the stairs, eager and anxious to practice under the watchful eye of the guru. For an Ashtangi, being in Mysore with Pattabhi is a true rite of passage. The yoga room only holds twelve people at a time, so one group of students will do their sun salutes and whatever series they're working on there, and then go upstairs to complete their finishing poses, including shoulderstand and headstand, making room for the next group to come in.

I wait an hour or so for my turn, watching through a small barred window, trying to get a sense of the protocol. I can see that the people around me are in awe, watching Pattabhi Jois closely. I watch him too. I keep waiting to feel some kind of illuminated vibration coming off him, something extraordinary, something divine. He's the guru, after all. But Pattabhi mostly sits on a stool in the corner of the room, clad in only Calvin Klein boxer briefs and a *yajnopavita*—a series of strings tied from his shoulder to the opposite hip representing the three gods: Brahma, Vishnu, and Shiva; the three sacrificial fires; the three divisions of time; and the three worlds. Every once in a while, he calls out an instruction in English, his accent thick, his tone impatient but not unkind. Sometimes he gets up, moves unsteadily across the overcrowded space, and makes a hands-on adjustment. Other times, he just leans against the wall and sleeps.

I hardly blame him for needing a nap. He's eighty-one years old after all and has been teaching round after round of students since 4 a.m.! His grandson, Sharath, does most of the work and is efficient, quiet, and professional. More often than not, when students have finished their practice upstairs, they come back into the room, kneel down before Pattabhi, thank him, and kiss the tops of his feet as a sign of respect.

Every day I watch through that window while I await my turn in the studio. It doesn't take long before I witness Pattabhi making adjustments I find unsettling. I wonder why his hand is where it is or why he seems to be moving his pelvis in kind of a creepy way. Before I came to India, I had heard others say, without elaborating, that his assists were "questionable," but I see nothing "questionable" about them. The way he touches some of the women—very differently from the way he touches the men—makes my alarm bells go off. In fact, there's no doubt in my mind that some of his adjustments are sexual in nature.

I spend a lot of time on those stairs reflecting on what I see. What if it happens to me? Would I leave? Would I freeze? Would I say something? Would I pretend nothing was happening? Would I simply endure it? Luckily, whenever I practice, Sharath seems to give me more attention than Pattabhi does. He's definitely very hands-on, but always appropriate and intentional. I never feel anything but deeply respected and safe with Sharath.

When I ask the other students if they think Pattabhi's adjustments are inappropriate, they tell me that Guruji would never be inappropriate, that he's only trying to help us go deeper. They say that the Guru doesn't have the same relationship with the human body as we do; if he happens to touch a student in an odd way, it's only because he's teaching them something they need to learn. Essentially I am told that it's no big deal; I should just get over it.

Then one day in the shala when I'm in Reclining Big-Toe Pose, Pattabhi comes over to me and lays his whole body over mine. I'm on the floor, on my back, and now completely trapped under his weight. He has one hand on my leg, pushing it down over my head, telling me to breathe, his face only inches from mine. My leg lowers effortlessly under his pressure, and he tells me, in a low gravelly voice, "Good, good." Then, gently but intentionally, he presses his penis against my vulva three times, his hips raising and lowering slowly against me.

I watch myself dissociate under the weight of his body, submitting to his assist. My mouth tightens into a thin line, but I say nothing.

Because I have already seen how he is with other female students, I'm not surprised when it happens to me. But I am saddened and disappointed that, once again, I cannot speak up. Every day during practice, I wait for him to approach me and wonder what the "assist" will be for that day. Boob grab? Ass squeeze? Vag pat? Or will I skate by with no grope at all? Oddly enough, the few times I've been in a room with him alone, he's been quiet, but kind, barely even making eye contact and certainly never touching me. His inconsistent behavior is confusing, but his actions in the shala are not.

Finally, one morning while I'm in a seated forward bend, Pattabhi comes up behind me and lays the full weight of his body onto my back, instructing me to breathe. He then proceeds to press his pelvis against my butt repeatedly. Once again, trapped under his weight, I can barely breathe. I feel his limp penis pushing against me. Finally, swatting him with my one free arm, I muster the courage to say, "Stop!" From across the room, Sharath begins speaking quickly and angrily to his grandfather in their native tongue. Pattabhi answers back, his tone equally quick and sharp. Then, slowly and awkwardly, he lifts himself off my body. I don't know what they said to one another, but I do know that for the rest of my stay in Mysore, Pattabhi never adjusts me again.

When I share my concerns again about Pattabhi's adjustments with some of the other more experienced students, they reply, with a knowing smile, that I had received an "initiation." I say, "An initiation? Are you out of your mind? Let's just call this what it is. If we choose to endure it, then that's on us, but let's not pretend this isn't actually happening!" No one is willing to go there. In fact, everyone I speak to seems to be in denial, a state I'm quite familiar with. This time, however, I know exactly what's going down, and I vow to stay present and be honest about all of it—even though the environment in Mysore is triggering for me and I should probably leave.

Pattabhi is not my guru. The more I learn about him, the more I understand his behavior, but still, I can never condone it. His elevated position and status have protected him from taking responsibility for the consequences of his actions. This is not unique to Pattabhi; this behavior plays out in yoga rooms all over the US.

Unless and until we commit to doing our own deep inner work, take responsibility for our woundedness, speak up, and hold each other accountable, I suspect this abuse of power will continue.

I cross Pattabhi Jois off my guru list.

I arrive in Pondicherry the day before the Mother's birthday. I go directly to the Matrimandir, a huge domelike temple that the Mother had been building prior to her death. Although the main chamber is still under construction, students are allowed in, to sit and meditate. I join the other visitors sitting in a circle on crisp, pristine cushions in the all-white room, in the center of which is a massive cut crystal. Directly above the crystal, at the top of the domed ceiling, is a small glass window. At certain times of the day, the sun shines through the small hole and onto the crystal; we happen to be there at one of those magical moments. Rainbow prisms of color shoot off the crystal and onto the walls, the floor, and our bodies. It is extraordinarily beautiful and peaceful. I lift my head toward the ceiling, open my eyes to the shimmering lights and my heart to the mystery of it all, and, as I often do in moments of true beauty, begin to quietly cry.

The next day I awake rejuvenated and affirmed. Something about this place speaks to me. I feel at home and at peace. Because it's the Mother's birthday, Pondicherrry has a huge celebration planned. Hundreds of thousands of people are expected to come and pay their respects at the Mother's *Mahasamadhi* (sometimes called *the Samadhi*), the shrine erected at her grave site, where her remains lay buried next to Sri Aurobindo's.

Being there on such an auspicious day makes me anxious. Only a couple of days earlier, I had left Pattabhi Jois's place and headed to see Mata Amritanandamayi Devi (Ammachi or Amma for short), a Hindu spiritual leader known as the hugging saint, also in Mysore, to receive *darshan*, the blessing offered by a holy person. Me and about thirty thousand other people. Her presence caused a mass frenzy, and I was almost trampled to death, literally, as throngs of people aggressively pushed forward toward a queue that began in a large field and funneled into a small gateway that could accommodate only one person at a time. At one point I was crushed between bodies so tightly that I was lifted off my feet and carried toward the gate. I was pretty certain that I would die that evening, crushed to death as I made my way to spiritual ecstasy! When I got to the small gateway, the male cops decided to block me by putting a wooden barricade between me and the entrance to Amma. I felt the force of thousands of people behind me pushing my chest into the barricade as I gasped for breath. I pleaded with the cops to open the gate, but they just ignored me. Finally, two female cops saw what was happening and pulled me through to safety. I dropped to my knees convinced I was about to faint. If I hadn't been so freaked out, I would've laughed when I saw one of the cops take off her shoe and swat the others with it until they told me they were sorry.

By the time I made it to Amma, I was anxious and overwhelmed. She hugged me, but I felt no relief. In the past, when I had visited her in the States, her embrace had left me feeling contented and connected. This time, I felt nothing. I tried to hug her back, feeling horrible that she had to deal with all this chaos day in and day out, but my arms were pushed away quickly by some unseen devotee. The whole scene wasn't going well for me. I had been pulled on stage to sit next to her, as another devotee tossed marigold and rose petals at me. I knew this was supposed to be a blessing and an honor, but I wasn't in the headspace for it at all. There was nothing special about me to warrant that honor, except that I was a white Westerner, which apparently afforded me some kind of elevated status. I sat there on the stage inches from the guru, comfortably isolated from the aggressive crowd. I picked the petals out of my hair and stared at the ground in front of me, trying to process what had happened, wondering why I was really there, and what I was supposed to learn from it all.

So now, the mere thought of hundreds of thousands of people descending upon Pondicherry fills me with dread. As I approach the Samadhi, I keep listening for the roar of people shouting and singing as they push their way to the front of the line. Instead, what I experience is something I will never forget. Sitting cross-legged and meditating quietly, thousands and thousands of people patiently wait their turn to inch forward toward the Mother's grave. It is so completely different from what I had experienced a few days earlier, a most magnificent sight. The power of presence, shared breath, and collective intention is palpable. If this is what happens when one is a disciple of Sri Aurobindo and the Mother, then I want in! I take my place in line, meditate, share food with those around me, and patiently wait my turn.

After many, many hours, I find myself close to the grave. I have been praying fervently all day, something I've never really done before. I have focused my attention on Sri Aurobindo, imploring him to show me God, and to help me feel God's presence within. I want guidance. I want illumination. I want to understand the ways of love. As I get close to the Samadhi, my prayers deepen. The energy coming off the grave is powerful; it's like a magnet pulling me toward it. I start feeling slightly dizzy and disembodied and experience a distinct buzzing sensation just under my skin. I am so present, open, and alive! I keep praying.

When it's finally my turn, I have to crawl toward the grave. My legs are too weak to carry me. I am filled with grace and awareness, certain I am home and with my true teachers. My heart is full to overflowing.

I get to the Samadhi, a large cement tomb with Sri Aurobindo entombed on one side and the Mother on the other. It is covered with thousands of beautiful flowers—marigolds, roses, and carnations—twelve inches deep at least. I am on my knees at Aurobindo's side, and I drop my face into the flowers, the scent intoxicating, and begin praying out loud.

"Dear God, open me, show me, and reveal to me your mystery, your light, your love. Sri Aurobindo, are you my guru? Should I leave home and live here to be closer to you? Please give me a sign, some direction so I know what to do, what to believe, how to surrender! Is it my will? Take it! Is it my ego? Take it! I want to be free, I want to heal, I want to know the God within, I want to experience real love. What should I do? Can you guide me? I want to know God! Show me God!"

Suddenly, I feel a sharp, intense bolt of energy, starting at my third eye and ripping down through my body. It is immediate, electrifying, hot, and sharp, and I gasp from the intensity of the sensation. Holy shit! It's Shaktipat! I had heard about this transmission of energy given from the master to the student. I had heard about its ecstasy and the waves of pleasure and openness you feel as you awaken to it. I had heard that it dissolves the illusion of separation and helps you experience the totality of Oneness!

The problem is I'm not feeling any pleasure or Oneness. Not even a little. My forehead is hot and painful, like it's burning from the inside. It's definitely real, though, and I don't want to miss one second of it. I keep breathing into the sensation as it pulses through my body, the intensity increasing. I keep waiting for the surge of ecstasy I am sure must be coming.

Instead, I hear a voice in my head say, *Fuck, this hurts!* Another voice interjects. *Breathe, take it in, let it fill you up.* I breathe. The first voice continues. *Maybe, but this fucking hurts!* It really does. The longer I stay with it, the worse it gets. Finally, I can't take the pain any longer, and I pull my head up off the flowers on the grave and put my hand on my third eye . . .

. . . and quickly remove the large bee that's been stinging me right between my brows.

You can imagine my disappointment.

I stay in Pondicherry for a couple more days. I try to read the *Savitri*, Sri Aurobindo's epic poem, under a grove of trees while bulldozers graze land for yet another shrine. I sit for hours with one of the main teachers and watch him flirt with a friend and make inappropriate advances. I walk the beach at the Bay of Bengal in the early morning and witness people going down to the shoreline and taking a shit, adding to the piles of shit everywhere. My enthusiasm evaporates. None of the guidance I craved or the deep teachings I longed for materialize and, once again, I feel disillusioned and alone. I go back to the Matrimandir to meditate. I sit in the main chamber and watch as the light hits the crystal and scatters rainbows everywhere, but now it all seems so contrived.

As I remain there, wallowing in my self-pity, my thoughts turn to Billy. I see him standing across the bar from me, a red ruby gleaming in his right ear. I see his smile, and I suddenly feel his love for me expand my own heart. I remember the last time he kissed my cheek and said goodbye, his smell a mixture of vetiver and decay. He removed the triangle necklace he was wearing and pressed it into my palm.

I sit up straight and feel his love rush in, as though he were there with me, in that moment, kissing my cheek, touching my hand. My body warms. I smile back at his invisible presence and feel him within me.

"Angels are everywhere, Seane. Every moment, every experience, in all beings, and in all time and space. That is where you will find God. Go within."

My eyeballs turn upward toward my third eye. The residual pain of the bee sting sharpens for a moment before the energy in my head expands. *"Go within,"* I hear Billy say again.

Everything becomes still. There's no sound, just a slight whooshing in my ears. No thoughts. No images. Nothing.

After a long while, I slowly open my eyes.

Shit. I don't need a guru. I don't need to search far and wide for something that's already within me. That's what Billy was trying to tell me all along, right? The teacher is in me and in you, in the easy times and the hard ones? In the heartbreak and in the beauty? I can almost see Billy nodding his head. Every experience is meant to awaken us to love and every person is the guru. Fuck, *life* is the guru! Each moment contains a message and offers significant guidance. I need to assign meaning, even to the incomprehensible. That is how I heal. That is how I love. That is how to know God. No, that is how to *be* God, by being love.

I begin to understand that I don't need to sit at the foot of a "realized" being to know God. Billy was my teacher; so were all the people at Heaven, as well as David Life and Sharon Gannon and everyone I met at Life Café, Integral Yoga, and YogaWorks. Every lover I have ever had, Amma and the thirty thousand people she hugged and the thousands paying their respects at the Samadhi. The Mother, my mother, my whole family. India, Pattabhi Jois, every stranger who has crossed my path, the people who have harmed me—my molesters, perpetrators, and harassers, even the shit on the beach. Everyone. Everything. We are in the Mystery together, learning, growing, changing, evolving, and every single moment supports our awakening. It doesn't always look that way, but it's all designed to shape and mature our soul. Each experience a teaching, every person a guru. All moments and all people hold a mirror up to us and reflect back those places within ourselves that are separate from our own light. Reclaim that light, and the essence of God is known.

I prayed for illumination, I prayed for guidance, I prayed to wake up, and my prayer was answered . . . in the form of a motherfucking bee. It doesn't get more real, or more holy, than that.

TEACHINGS FROM INDIA
CLARITY, CONFIDENCE, AND THE GURU WITHIN

My friends convinced me that only a guru could initiate me into the mysteries of the heart and set me on the path toward enlightenment or bliss. That was the goal, right? Enlightenment. The result of all my hard work and practice. I wanted that. Who cares that the journey is the destination, that there isn't a goal in yoga, that yoga is now? All I knew was that I'd been busting my ass in this practice, and I wanted something more to show for it other than fabulous triceps.

The guru-student relationship, Paramahansa Yogananda once said, is the highest expression of friendship. But, he also said that gurus, often called the "dispellers of darkness," were the only ones who could lead seekers "on their inward journey toward perfection." To know God, you must find someone who is "God-realized," he wrote, who will tell you what to do, what to think, and how to live your life in accordance with God's principles. Students asked questions; gurus gave answers. Students

were seekers; gurus had sought and found. Students were asked to surrender their will to the guru, to give the guru unconditional devotion and unquestioned loyalty; gurus promised to give Shaktipat in return, a transmission of holy energy, which would awaken the Divine within the student. Only through the guru could students experience the true power of God. Didn't sound like a relationship to me.

Of course I realize that for millennia, the guru-disciple relationship has been a positive and necessary one for many practitioners, part of the ancient tradition of yoga and the culture from which it arose. And it's not like I had never met teachers I resonated with. I've definitely known truly enlightened masters in my life. People who carry with them a certain magic and an abundance of love. They have an ability to simply "be," and they possess a wisdom that is truly otherworldly. I've learned from them, and they've helped me along my path, but not once did they ask me to follow them. Nor did they ever suggest that they were the only extraordinary ones. Always, they inferred, what was within them radiates in all, and they reflected back to me the light within me that was waiting for recognition.

But when my friends first told me I needed a guru, I wasn't so sure. And for good reason. For one thing, the guru-student relationship is rooted in Indian culture, a culture quite different from my own. For another, I was judging it based on how it's been interpreted in the West—in US ashrams, spiritual communities, and even yoga studios—an interpretation I found deeply troubling. So, I figured that if I wanted to find a guru, transcend my ego, and know God, I needed to get to India.

WHEN YOU MEET THE BUDDHA

A huge stumbling block in my search for a teacher was the imbalance of power inherent in such a relationship, one which enforces within the student a belief that, without the guru's guidance, they can never know God. This power dynamic can be seductive for both the student *and* the guru. We've all seen far too many examples of gurus using their position of authority to dominate others, gurus who believe their own hype, and gurus who fall hard when they get caught with their pants down. It takes a strong sense of self and purpose to transcend the ego, to not mistake devotion for sexual attraction, and to not take advantage of weakness or insecurity.

As students, when we don't address our unhealed woundedness or low self-esteem, we look outside ourselves for validation, approval, and even love. It happens in our emotional-sexual relationships, in our family dynamics, and in many other aspects of our lives. Why wouldn't it also happen in guru-student relationships, especially when we are told that only the guru holds the key to our healing, that only the guru can bring peace to our soul?

I certainly wouldn't suggest that everyone abandon their teachers and strike out on their own. But I do suggest that if you decide to enter into a relationship with a guru, you do it with eyes wide open. It's too easy to slip into a codependency that doesn't serve your quest for spiritual awakening. I see this a lot in the Western yoga community, where regular yoga teachers have elevated themselves (with the help of their students) into exalted beings, lineage holders of deep truths. I've seen these teachers take advantage of students who seek their love and approval, exploiting their trust and diminishing their capacity to make their own life decisions and come to their own spiritual conclusions. It's never okay for a teacher to coerce you into doing anything you feel compromises you in any way—no matter how "touched by God" they are. If, at any time, the behavior of the guru you're with seems confusing or makes you uncomfortable, find a new teacher (if that is your path) or discover a new path to God. Remember, God lives within you, and you may not need a guru to discover that. But, as they say: many rivers, one ocean.

There's a saying in Buddhism that I love: "If you meet the Buddha, kill the Buddha." Obviously, it's symbolic. But what I get out of it is that the Buddha represents the image of the perfect teacher—the guru I so hoped to find. At first, I had to kill the idea that this guru must look or teach or act a certain way. In the end, I realized I had to kill the idea that the teacher is somehow separate from myself and could provide the awakening I was seeking. There is no separation between ourselves and God, between the mundane and the Divine. Everything lives within us. And teachers are everywhere. The moment you think you've found the one-and-only teacher or understand enlightenment, you're wrong! Kill that idea and keep practicing.

I went to India to meet my guru, and I came home empty-handed, yet fullhearted. Although not my guru in any traditional sense, each of the teachers I met was significant—because each one taught me the lesson I needed to learn, whether they realized it or not. I went to India prepared to give my power away; I came home with it fully intact and with a confidence I had lost long ago. I went to India to receive the blessing of the guru; I discovered the clarity of my own mind instead. I went to India as a seeker, searching for God outside of myself, but when I opened my heart, I saw that God was already there and had never been lost to me. I had been seeking what had already been found. It took the sting of a bee to penetrate my self-doubt and longing, to wake me up to my true nature, and to rekindle my confidence, clarity, and compassion. But first I had to systematically "meet the Buddha" and then "kill the Buddha."

THE BODY NEVER LIES: GAINING CONFIDENCE

I traveled to Mysore (now called Mysuru) thinking Pattabhi Jois was a true guru, an enlightened master. My mind was ready and eager to say yes. My body was not. And my body was right. My mind wanted to believe that Pattabhi was the one. People I loved and trusted told me he was, and the experiences they shared with me affirmed that. But the visceral reaction I had watching his behavior through the window on the stairs—even before he laid a hand on me—told another story. My body knew: he was not safe.

Asana practice, when it employs the breath and the mind, cultivates self-awareness, a sense of inner knowing. Every pose invites you to observe your reaction to it—does the pose feel spacious, steady, appropriate? Does it allow the breath to be smooth and long? Does it bring a sense of ease or even joy to the mind? Can you stay with the sensation? If not, how can you adjust, find a more appropriate response or a different expression of the pose itself? Of course, insights like these go beyond the yoga mat as you face challenging situations in real life. Does a certain experience cause you to contract? Do you find yourself holding your breath? What visceral sensation are you experiencing? Can you focus, be steady, open, flexible, present, and nonreactive, or do you want to run? When Pattabhi laid his body on top of mine the first time, my body recoiled, sending urgent, red-flag messages to my mind. Nothing about the experience was spacious, steady, or easeful. And it certainly wasn't joyful. And yet I didn't do anything to change it. Old traumas and old patterns resurfaced, and once again, I dissociated.

I was beginning to understand that the universe sends us the same lesson, in different guises, again and again, until we learn from it, heal, and grow. This time the universe sent me Pattabhi. And this time, I chose to stay present to what was happening, and I was prepared to take action. It didn't happen the first time or the second or the third, but when he touched me inappropriately the fourth time, I finally said, "Stop." And he stopped. In that moment I broke a pattern and began to call my power back.

Pattabhi Jois was a stark reminder of my childhood trauma and an embodiment of all the men who had accosted me and robbed me of my voice and my agency. And yet, he was also an important guide for me on my path to healing. How was that possible? Because, much like the bee that lodged in my forehead at the Mother's Mahasamadhi, Pattabhi stung me into action. He woke me up, and I had to take ownership of what was happening and not make excuses or shut down. He made me realize that failing to act was no longer an option. That I had control over my body and a responsibility to protect it at all costs. His actions empowered me to take a stand, to trust my intuition, and to know, with all my being, that what I had seen and experienced was exactly what had gone down. I didn't imagine it. I wasn't making it up. And I certainly wasn't making excuses for his behaviors. Pattabhi's shadow self met my own. His behaviors brought my shadow reactions to the surface. I saw them, I met them, I responded to them, and, in doing so, I found my voice, and I felt its power. As a result, I discovered the confidence I needed to confront injustice and break the pattern of harassment that often left me frozen and silent in fear and shame.

It wasn't a complete victory though. My time with Pattabhi also made me realize I had more work to do.

Remaining in a potentially harmful environment, instead of leaving, can show us where we're still a bit too willing to compromise ourselves. In my case, I wanted to be a part of the Mysore community, even though it also meant participating in a culture of secrecy. I still see my experience as an important step on my path toward untying the bonds that had held me captive for so long.

A MIND ENGAGED: FINDING CLARITY

I thought a quick detour to see Ammachi while she was in Mysore would move me to follow her. I was ready to melt into her embrace and receive darshan. Not this time, though. Instead, I nearly got trampled to death as thousands of devotees funneled into a single queue, nailing me to a wooden barricade, the one thing that separated them from their guru. It was frightening, chaotic, and disempowering—all of us jockeying for position, trying to get our piece of the spiritual pie, stepping on each other along the way. By the time I passed through the gate, my entire nervous system was shot. Although I knew in my heart, it wasn't Amma's fault—she's a remarkable woman, humanitarian, and teacher—the whole experience left me feeling anxious and overwhelmed. If this was what it was like being a devotee of Amma, I wanted nothing to do with it.

Nevertheless, Ammachi proved to be an important teacher for me. My interactions with the crowd, the bodyguards, and Amma herself gave me profound insight into my own mind—with all its judgments and misperceptions, arrogance and privilege. I projected everything I felt onto Amma and her followers—my irritation, my helplessness, and my overwhelm. I was freaked out, so obviously she must be too. I found myself thinking that I would protect her from the masses; I would fix everything by giving her the energy she needs to keep going. It never dawned on me that she might not feel the same as I did. Who the hell was I to presume I knew how she felt or what she thought? These people were *her* people, *her* followers; they were in *her* domain. I was the outsider, not them. And I was stuck in my presumptuous, judgmental mind.

What is this mind that jumps to conclusions when you're uncomfortable, when you're in a situation you can't comprehend or control? It's the manomaya kosha once again, the thinking mind that refuses to quiet down long enough for you to process what's really happening. The mind that sees or experiences something and makes a split-second decision to act, without understanding that its actions are clouded by preconceived judgments, cultural stigmas, hidden traumas, and repressed emotions. As long as your nervous system is destabilized and you're in fight-flight-freeze-fold mode, the mind remains in a fog. You can purify the mind and lift the confusion by engaging the wisdom mind, the vijnanamaya kosha—but it takes conscious breathing and meditative practices to make that commitment. From within this realm, you can see what is clinging to your muddled mind that prevents you from living with compassion and integrity. You can declutter it by noticing and releasing whatever is getting in your way—the judgments, past experiences, excuses, and fears. Calm, steady breathing creates a calm, steady mind, which helps you cultivate ahimsa (non-harming, non-judgment, love) and be present to whatever is going on around you and within you.

When Amma's handlers pulled me up on stage, I was relieved and certainly in no hurry to return to the maddening crowd. I was happy to have space to breathe and a spot away from the chaos. But my bee-sting moment came as I suddenly realized why I had been chosen out of the thousands who clamored for her attention, and my relief turned to disgust. I was on that stage for no other reason than the whiteness of my skin and the power that being a Westerner bestowed. That privilege entitled me the honor and the luxury of a front-row seat to the Divine and separated me from the rest of humanity that afternoon. If I had any doubts about any of this, all I had to do was look around me—every other person on that stage looked like me.

I got a taste of how this privilege, and the power dynamics that came with it, gave me advantages that kept me separate from the others. David had tried to teach me this at Life Café years before—but I didn't get it then. Now I saw it, and it could not have been clearer. This separation is endemic in our society; it perpetuates the oppression that harms and impedes certain groups while protecting and advancing others—based on race, religion, gender, sexuality, class, ability, and education—and it runs deep in the collective psyche, influencing how we experience ourselves and each other. This separation, the opposite of yoga, was alive and well—even in a yoga ashram, even in the lap of the guru. Throughout the world and in every culture, separation begets pain and suffering, which are the roots of all oppression.

I learned some invaluable lessons that day, and everyone there—Amma, the cops, and the crowd—were all my teachers. They and their actions were inviting me to witness the ways in which I unwittingly participated in this separation and benefited from it.

I wanted clarity, and that is exactly what I got. This insight set me on a path of personal and cultural investigation, which in the years to come would greatly impact my spiritual development and my commitment to activism and service. Amma was not my guru in any traditional sense but, like Pattabhi, she was another teacher and proved to be an important guide on my path.

AN EXPANDED HEART: FEELING COMPASSION

By the time I left Mysore, I was feeling pretty discouraged. But then, I arrived in Pondicherry (now called Puducherry). Whoa, I thought, this is it. It was everything I had craved. I felt like I was in Xanadu. Just like being in a great cathedral, it was all so inspiring. God *must* be here, right? It was too heavenly for anything other than the Divine. Its orderliness and its elegance were outward manifestations of all things transcendent, I just knew it.

Wait a sec. Wasn't I first introduced to God in a sex club? And in the grit and the grime of New York City's Lower East Side? Clearly, I needed a reality check. What made me think God had suddenly decided that crystals and rainbows and disciples decked out in white were the only suitable trappings for Divine presence? Just because my experiences in Mysore made *me* uncomfortable didn't mean that God wasn't there. God was everywhere, in everyone and everything, as Billy taught me, but I didn't see it, and I didn't feel it until I got to Pondicherry—or so I thought. But Pondicherry wasn't everywhere and everything either, not by a long shot.

So what the hell was happening? I had thought that India would provide the guru I needed to liberate me from my shadow self, to set me on a path toward enlightenment. I was determined to find my teacher. This singleness of purpose, this intense focus, is tapas. I just knew if I prayed more, worked harder, kept searching, I'd find the One. I somehow missed the memo that tapas is not an outward-driven practice; it's an inward investigation. I also seemed to forget that I had agency, that I got to decide what worked best for my own journey toward liberation. That's svadhyaya—the capacity to see what's true in every moment, to distinguish what we really need from what others tell us we need or what we think we ought to need.

And finally, I discovered what happens when I choose to move out of my small self and see the Divine in all beings. I found God not in the shala of Pattabhi Jois, in the hugs of Ammachi, or in the rainbows and flowers of Pondicherry, but within myself. Yogis call this ishvara pranidhana—radical openness, surrender, devotion, communion with the Divine—the fifth of the five niyamas. When that happened, I witnessed the sacredness of the whole world. Swami Satchidananda nailed it when he said we must surrender to what *is*, which "requires trust in our deepest Self, our intuition and the courage to express ourselves for who we are, as we are, with all of our perfect imperfections, all of which ultimately leads to freedom."

It took a bee sting to get my attention. There I was on my knees, praying for an awakening, asking to be shown the way, the light. But when I discovered a bee drilling a small hole in my forehead, I prayed instead that I wouldn't end up going into anaphylactic shock. I felt teased. I wanted my awakening to be joyful, pleasurable, and ecstatic. Instead it was painful, disappointing, and ordinary. But isn't that life? Doesn't life hold all of it? Doesn't the shadow reveal the light? Isn't there beauty even in the grotesque, magic even in the mundane?

I certainly wasn't ready to concede that lesson.

All along, I looked for answers and guidance from everyone and everything outside of myself. I was willing to give my power away and to deny an authentic relationship with Source—unless it was first affirmed by someone else . . . or unless it felt pleasurable or ecstatic. And then that bee stopped me in my tracks. As it pierced my third eye, my realization was swift and sharp: No matter how hard I tried, how long I searched, or how far I traveled, I would never find my guru. Because there *was* no guru for me to find. As I walked around Pondicherry, I felt its magic dissolve, its gold become tarnished, and its glitter dimmed. Maybe it was me. Maybe the bloom was off the rose simply because I hadn't gotten what I came for. As a white Western yoga seeker, I expected India to be my everything. I wanted to see rainbows and crystals and the power of God everywhere. All my friends said India changed their lives; why hadn't it changed mine? Or had it?

I suddenly saw how willing I was to believe what I wanted so badly to believe, and how willing I was to judge things when they failed to live up to my expectations. I came to Pondicherry ready to open my heart and feel connected to God and to all beings, and instead I was about to leave feeling judgy, disappointed, and sad. But then, I sat down and closed my eyes, my forehead still throbbing from the bee sting, which clearly had more to teach me. I was ready to listen.

If there is no guru outside of myself, who will guide me? That blessed sting seemed to say stop searching and you will find the answer. Teachers and angels are everywhere, even in a big patch of flowers; the guru I was seeking had been within me all along. God was also in everything and in everybody and in all moments. The beautiful ones, the boring ones, the grief-filled ones, and even the tragic ones. There is not a single moment that is not of God, and every moment, all experiences, are meant to awaken us to this knowing and open our hearts in empathy and compassion. Even my experiences in India. They had played out exactly as they were supposed to for the evolution of my soul. Hell yeah, they were painful, confusing, and hard. But they sure as hell woke me up and even brought me a little closer to my true nature.

I left India without a guru but came home with something infinitely more powerful: confidence, clarity, and compassion. Whether they knew it or not, the teachers I met gave me what I had prayed for most of my adult life—the confidence to heed my body's wisdom, the clarity to trust my intuition, and the compassion to love without exception. I felt love for the whole world, for the bitter, beautiful, glorious, tragic, and wondrous mystery of it all, and, for the first time, I knew without a doubt that the "heaven" I had been seeking was right here all along—everywhere I look and wherever I am.

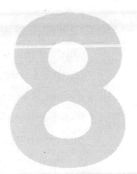

SAY HIS NAME, BABY

I RETURNED FROM INDIA with a new-found confidence—on and off my mat. I was happy simply to roll out my mat and move in synchronicity with my deep breaths. I particularly loved practicing vinyasa flow. *Vinyasa*, which means "to place in a special way," links movement with breath. It's rhythmic, informed by proper alignment, and, because it's not attached to any particular school of yoga, spiritually open to personal interpretation. Through the freedom and independence of vinyasa, I felt like I was integrating all I had learned from my many teachers, and my practice was becoming more personal, creative, embodied, and present. I began teaching—after lots of trainings and mentorships—and I was finally able to experience longer periods of deep stillness on my mat, on my cushion, and in my life. I was confident that I had the skills to ground myself and the emotional integration I needed to weather just about any conflict or crisis that arose. And then I got my heart broken . . .

My boyfriend and I had been together for five years, and I treasured our life together. I was deeply in love. We shared so many of the same interests and felt at ease and at home with each other. I valued and honored our connection and did everything I could to protect it, and so did he. Or so I thought.

A couple of years after I got back from India, we started having some challenges. Our communication wasn't as fluid. Our arguments took longer to resolve. The tension between us resulted in bouts of silence and hurt feelings. As he became more distant, I became more desperate, trying to get him to engage. It was tiresome, but it didn't feel dire. I was still confident about our commitment—to each other and to our relationship.

Then, late one night when we were both asleep, he rolled over on top of me and awakened me with an intense and passionate kiss. I felt the weight of his body on me, his hands in my hair, but before I had a chance to respond, he rolled off, turned over onto his side, away from me, and continued to snore lightly. I whispered his name, but he didn't respond. He was very much asleep. I lay there on my back, staring up at the ceiling. I should have felt the excitement of that spontaneous moment, a rush of erotic energy, the desire to finish what he had started. But I didn't. Instead, the deep clarity of what I suddenly knew to be true caused my body to tremble and the tears began to flow.

That was not my kiss. It did not belong to me. I knew with absolute certainty that the man I loved was seeing someone else, that my relationship was unraveling, and that my world was about to shift in a way I did not welcome.

The next morning, I asked if he remembered kissing me. He said he didn't. I described what happened, but he just laughed, shook his head, and passed it off as nothing. I tried to ground myself and remain calm, but inside I was shaking, and my heart was beating wildly. Everything in my body told me that he was no longer present in this relationship. I wanted confirmation, but I already knew the truth.

So, my eyes locked on his, I asked him if he was having an affair.

He looked at me for the longest time, bewildered and confused. "No," he said. "Why would you even suggest that?"

"Because that was not my kiss," I said. "That was for someone else. I have absolutely no doubt about it, but I need you to tell me the truth."

He laughed and rolled his eyes in exasperation, as though I was forever taunting him with accusations of infidelity, which I was not.

"Please tell me."

"Seane, I was sleeping. I didn't do anything wrong. I don't remember anything. It was just a kiss! Absolutely nothing is going on. I swear. I promise."

I stood there looking into his eyes for evidence to the contrary. He stared back at me, insulted that I would even suggest something like that. I told him that I didn't believe him, that I knew in my gut he was lying. He told me to stop. How could I accuse him of such a thing? How could I devalue our relationship like that? I felt my resolve slip.

Still, I asked him one more time. "Please tell me the truth. Everything in my body says you are lying. Tell me I'm not crazy."

"Seane," he said, as he placed his hands gently on my shoulders, "Nothing's going on. You're completely making this up. It's all in your head. You *are* crazy."

I felt foolish and ashamed. Am I really that insecure, that fearful? It's certainly not in my nature to be jealous or suspicious. But is that what I'm being? Why do I keep badgering him when he told me I was wrong the first time? Why can't I just let it go? Obviously this was my shit—old abandonment crap I hadn't fully dealt with and was projecting on him. And what other evidence did I have but a kiss he gave me in his sleep?

But, if he *was* telling me the truth, what did that say about my intuition, which had guided me and long been my source of truth? How could I have been so off? When did my body start to lie to me? What else was I wrong about?

As a sensitive child, I could easily intuit when something wasn't right, even if the evidence suggested otherwise. Often what I "knew" didn't match what I was being told. My head, heart, and body said one thing, but others insisted on something else entirely and let me know, in no uncertain terms, that I was wrong. That confused me, but being so young, I didn't have words to describe my confusion. I had no way to explain why I knew what I knew was true. Instead I'd get frustrated, angry, and rail against injustice—against me, against my friends, and against the world. These big feelings—and the aggressive way I expressed myself—proved to others that I was emotional and "crazy," an assessment they weren't shy about handing down. An assessment that made me question—and at times distrust—my inner knowing.

It took years of doing yoga and inner work before I could listen to the messages of my body and have confidence in my intuitive nature once again. But the moment the man I loved called me "crazy," all of that dissolved, and I spiraled back to the small place within me that whispered: *Perhaps he's right. Perhaps they're all right. I'm just nuts.*

So, I apologized.

Of course, as it turned out, I *was* right. And he was 100 percent full of shit. He had been lying and totally having an affair. We broke up.

Our breakup devastated me. It didn't matter that what he did was awful and that I didn't want to be with a liar and a cheat. Intellectually, I knew I was better off without him. But emotionally? I was a wreck. I couldn't sleep or eat or think of anything other than him, us, and the how, when, why of it all. My every nerve felt inflamed. I went to sleep crying; I woke up crying. I was utterly heartbroken. I felt betrayed and abandoned and resented the hell out of him. And yet, I ached for him in ways I could never have imagined. I missed his smell, his touch, his very presence in my life. I didn't even know how to begin to disentangle myself from him. I felt him in my body, in every room of our once-shared home, in our cats, which, like me, he left behind. The breakup brought up all my attachment issues. It's always been hard enough for me to let go of the inanimate objects I love, so you can imagine how I felt losing the love of my life so abruptly. I missed him terribly and was disgusted at myself for it.

I knew this breakup had brought up some deep feelings of abandonment, but I couldn't believe that the tools that I had counted on for years—my yoga and meditation practice—had deserted me as well. I slipped into my old familiar patterning to self-soothe, which left the bottoms of my feet—once a target of my anxiety—cut, peeled, and torn. I was deeply depressed—a state of being I'd never experienced before. No amount of yoga offered me relief. Every breath I took got lodged in my throat. I would sometimes get through a few minutes of asana, but then fatigue would take over, and I would lie in Child's Pose, unable to move. Nothing I did eased my pain. I obviously needed help.

One morning, the phone rang. I picked it up and, through my tears, managed a feeble "Hello . . . ?"

Marti was on the other line. A longtime friend, who often called me in the morning to check in, she could hear the pain in my voice. "Oh Seanie," she said. "Go ahead and let all those tears out. But you won't be able to see the truth of this until you get the anger out too." I cried harder. "Go see Mona," Marti said. "She's my, ummm, therapist. Yeah, I guess you could call her that. No matter, she's brilliant and spot-on, but also kinda out of her mind . . . in a really good way. I promise, you'll adore her. She's intense, and a little quirky, but she'll walk you through this."

Quirky? I hadn't a clue what she meant by that, but I was pretty sure it didn't matter what she was, as long as she could help me.

I called Mona and left her a message, explaining briefly what was going on and telling her I needed an appointment. An hour later, the phone rang. I picked it up and heard a cheerful, high-pitched, childlike voice on the other end say, "Hi baby, tell me what's going on!" as if she was my closest girlfriend returning my call. I babbled on about my breakup and the betrayal I felt. She listened, throwing in a "that motherfucker!" here and there—which I appreciated in a girl-to-girl kind of way; I did find it a bit odd though that a therapist would support my judgments so enthusiastically. Finally, interrupting my diatribe, she said, "Honey, you're totally fucked up right now, and for good reason. Why don't you get in your car, come over, and let's see if we can rinse this shit from you. Then we can really talk."

Rinse this shit? "Okay. I'm coming over."

▼

I have no trouble finding Mona's house because it's awash in Halloween decorations. I don't mean a carved pumpkin on the stoop and a few bats hanging from the trees. I mean every square inch of land and home is covered by store-bought ghosts, goblins, witches, black cats, flashing lights, you name it. Walking up the pathway to the front door, I'm greeted by animated murderous ghouls set off by unseen sensors, whose open-mouthed screams and shrills make me jump. I consider going home immediately.

The door is open, so I step inside. The nightmare of Walmart-purchased Halloween horror continues unabated with decorations, lights, and streamers everywhere. The screaming from outside echoes through the house itself.

I look around in disbelief. Marti calls this woman quirky? I think she's fucking nuts. Her preteen son comes out of some back room, walks into the kitchen, says hi, and asks if I want some water. He looks normal enough, I think, but how does he deal with the constant yelling coming out of the mouths of those animated ghouls?

"Fuck you!" I hear a scream from somewhere upstairs and then, "I fucking hate you!" which seems to come from behind the door nearby. What the hell? That can't be the decorations. I listen some more and realize that the yelling is coming from real people somewhere in this house.

"Fuck you, Mom!" "I hate you, Dad!" "Motherfucker, asshole, dick-eating, cunt, whore!"

I glance at Mona's son, who's making a sandwich. He looks at me, smiles and shrugs, and goes back into his room.

Who are these people? Why are they here, and why are they yelling like this? I take a fistful of candy corns from a bowl and shove them in my mouth as I survey the scene. In the room off the kitchen, where a dining room should be, is an all-white room (minus the Halloween decorations, of course), where a white baby grand piano sits in one corner surrounded by several small white tables and chairs, like a nightclub. Strewn across the piano is a hot-pink feather boa and pages and pages of sheet music. The rest of the house is filled to the brim with furniture, paintings, and knickknacks that are lacquered, overstuffed, colorful, whimsical, and mismatched. To say it was a bit much would be a ridiculous understatement.

Suddenly Mona bounds down the stairs to greet me. "Seane!" she says and walks over to me, grabs me hard, and hugs me to her chest as if she hasn't seen me in years when, in fact, we've never met before. She releases me, holds me at arm's length, stares into my eyes, and squints.

After a moment she chirps, "Oh, he's really fucked you up, hasn't he? No matter." Her bright-blue eyes are twinkling, "You'll thank him one day. You really will. But not yet. Right now, you're hurt, and you feel like your life is a shitshow, so let's get this crap out of you so we can get down to the truth!"

She grabs my hand and leads me up the stairs. I use this moment to take her in. Her hair is curly and bright blonde, a little over-bleached at the ends. She's wearing hot-pink sweatpants and a tight white T-shirt with a heart covered in pink rhinestones and *L-O-V-E* spelled out across her boobs, which are pretty impressive. She's also wearing thick fuzzy purple socks and is adorned in bracelets, necklaces, and rings. Not flashy jewelry, just a lot of it. I guess her to be in her late thirties. She's quite pretty, very charismatic, excessively cheerful, and looks as bright and animated as a cartoon character. She matches her house perfectly.

As I reach the top of the stairs, the yelling gets louder. A pounding noise adds to the cacophony. I could swear it's coming from the closet nearby, and I hesitate.

Mona glances my way and says, "That's called anger work. People come over when they need to rinse out their big feelings. Just ignore it. They're doing their thing and working it out. They're fine."

I now hear someone howling and crying from inside the closet. Mona knocks on the door and says, "You fine?" "Fine!" the person replies and then continues to pound on something and shout, "Fuck you, you motherfucking piece of shit!"

Mona smiles and says, "See!" and, still holding my hand, leads me to a back room.

The room is a whole 'nother level of strange. There's a large, velvet, multicolored, round couch-bed-thing she instructs me to sit on. Paintings, stuffed animals, books, and papers are everywhere. "This looks like the playroom for a twelve-year-old child," I tell her, "not a therapist's office."

Mona bursts out laughing. "Oh sweetheart, I am not a therapist! I'd be thrown in jail for the shit I do if I were! Nope," she says, "I'm more of a life coach, best friend, communication expert, channel, and all-around fuck-your-shit-up kind of gal. Now tell me. What's up, oh Vibeless One?"

Vibeless One? Suddenly I feel overwhelmed, so I take a breath, sit up straight, and put my feet on the floor. I need to get back in my body. I take another deep breath and start to explain my relationship and the betrayal I feel, not only because he cheated, but because he made me believe I was crazy. I go on and on, feeling really good about how honest and self-aware I am being. I explain that I don't want to throw him under the bus. That I'm ready to take some responsibility for the relationship ending, definitely willing to look at my part in all of it, especially my codependency. I'm pretty sure, I say, that I gave my power away and that there are important spiritual lessons in this, which are meant to help me grow. I'm sure we were in each other's life to teach one another important lessons. I mean, right? I tell her the whole story and end by saying I am really hurt, angry, and sad.

"Oh. Really? You're sad? You don't seem terribly sad. How do you feel right now?"

"I don't know. Right now?" I think about it for a second. "Fine, I guess."

Mona laughs. "You know what *F-I-N-E* means? Fucked up, insecure, neurotic, and emotional!"

I stare at her.

"So do you think you're crazy?" she asks.

"Fuck no!" I say. "He said I was crazy; I don't think I'm crazy at all. He was trying to make me believe I was though."

"And you did?"

"Yes. I totally thought I was making it up. I felt like such an idiot."

"Where did you learn that was true?"

"What? Being crazy or being an idiot?"

"Both."

"I don't know—I guess when I was young, I got told that a lot."

"Really? Who told you that? How old were you?"

I try answering her questions, telling her that I used to have "gut feelings" about what was going on around me, but whenever I tried to share them, I was told they weren't true; I was told I was mistaken. That often made me second-guess myself. When that happened, I'd get so frustrated, I'd rage.

"What would happen when you raged?"

"I'd be told to shut up, or I'd be laughed at. Sometimes, if I got really out of control, my father might smack me."

"So you learned that raging was bad and that it was safer to suppress your big feelings?"

I can't speak; it feels like something is caught in my throat. So I nod my head.

Mona takes a sip from the 32-ounce Coca-Cola she's nursing and says, "Honey, you're not crazy, but you have voices in your head that are, and they have been with you a long time, way before you met that guy. They are part of your shadow self. Do you know about the shadow?" I nodded my head again.

"Good. Then we've got to go get 'em. Right now, your ego is blocking you from seeing the truth. You need to understand what the ego is trying to teach you, in the same way you need to understand what your ex was here to teach you.

There's something way bigger going on, and he's only a small piece of it. Actually, my love, he's your angel . . ."

"No, he's not!" I say, outraged that she would even suggest that this lying, cheating motherfucker was somehow instrumental to my growth. I surprise myself with the intensity of my reaction. I got triggered. I relax my balled-up fists and take a breath. My ego was up; she's right. All I have is my judgment to cling to, and it's got way more power than my love. Fuck. This is going to be hard.

"Relax, it's true . . ." She squints at me again and continues, "But you already know that. Not only is he your teacher, but remember what I said, one day you'll thank him. But not yet. This is a God thing not a relationship thing. You prayed for this, Seane; you hear me? You did this. It's not personal, it's spiritual . . . and it's the gift that will bring you back to yourself. He is just holding the mirror up to show you the ways you've been disconnected from your highest Self."

Mona puts down her Coke and, looking very pleased with herself, shoves some kind of hard candy in her mouth, and waits for me to say something.

I just stare. Breathing deeply in and out, I try to stay calm. My body feels thick and tingly, and the more she speaks, the more lightheaded I feel, as energy swirls around my head.

Suddenly Mona raises her arm and waves her hand in front of my face.

"Hello!" She says calmly, "Where'd you go? Are you here? Are you in your body right now?"

Startled, I shake my head. "Huh?"

"Sweetheart, you're dissociating. You're in your shutdown. That's why I called you vibeless. Lights on, nobody home!" She waves a hand across my face once again.

Now I'm annoyed, but I show no emotion. She smiles and says, half-kiddingly, "You yogis are the worst to work with! Detachment, right? That's what you strive for, isn't it? Well, let me tell you something, Yogi. Detachment without true awareness is just dissociation, and it's something I have no doubt you are brilliant at. You've gotten really good at understanding your pain; you can even articulate it beautifully, but you suck balls at actually feeling it. That's true, isn't it?"

I sit there, wide-eyed, my heart beating fast. It is true. I could *explain* how I felt, but I couldn't always *feel* what I felt. But I had felt my emotions, that day in

Bryan's class, hadn't I? I had learned to be present to what came up, allow it to surface, witness it, and then let it go. So, I have no idea what she wants from me, but whatever it is, I'm not sure I want to deliver it. I want to run. I feel exposed. I suddenly realize that Mona is about to ask me to *feel* my feelings fully, to enter into my pain, in ways I have never done before—and frankly, have never wanted to.

"So how do you feel?" she asks.

"I don't know . . . freaked out, I guess." My breath is coming in and out, short and controlled. I look at her helplessly and say, "I just feel so empty."

She leans forward and takes one of my feet in her hands, looks at the bandages, and raises an eyebrow in question. I look down at the floor. She begins to massage it gently. "You're not empty, baby. Actually, you're full. You're full of anger, fear, rage, shame, guilt, jealousy, disappointment, and grief, and you're taking it out on your poor feet and who knows what else. It's all old shit. And it's all too much. So, you go into shutdown as a way to protect. This is how you've survived the overwhelm you felt as a kid, but it doesn't work anymore. You need to let your crazy voices speak. You need to give your little girl permission to fully air out and say everything she needs to—from her gut, without intellectualizing. That's the only way we can get to the truth. How does that sound?"

Not waiting for an answer, she gets up, her rhinestone bracelets jingling as she removes them from her wrist. She takes off her shiny rings and then, reaching behind the chair, pulls out a tennis racket and a foam cushion.

She then shouts some woman's name and asks her to come into the room. The young woman in the hallway closet emerges—I'll call her Lisa—her eyes bright red and swollen from crying, her hair a big mess. Mona introduces us. I awkwardly go to shake her hand. She puts it in the air and says, "Sorry, can't touch you, too much snot." She and Mona laugh, and Mona hands her a tissue. That's when I notice there are boxes of tissues everywhere.

Mona gives me a brief rundown on Lisa's story: Recovered alcoholic. Three years in juvie. Sexually molested by step-brother and cousin. Mad Internet skills, and if you ever need help on the computer, she's your girl.

Why am I privy to all of this, I wonder? This isn't my business. It strikes me as odd that Mona would so casually share this person's story with me, a complete stranger—when she's standing right there!

As though she could read my mind, Mona interrupts my train of thought, smiles, and says, "We break shame around here. This is all about normalizing the human experience—that means we *own* truth, even if it's an ugly truth. Better out than in!"

She turns back to Lisa and says, "Seane just had her heart ripped out by the man she loves and is in shutdown out of low ego and self-protection. She can *admit* her feelings, but she needs to own them. Show her how it's done."

With that, Lisa drops to her knees, draws the tennis racket over her head, and starts beating the cushion. "Fuck you, motherfucker! Fuck you! I was just a little girl! A beautiful, innocent child!" She stops, takes a breath, and then pounds the cushion some more. She continues hitting it and screaming profanities. Mona then offers prompts. "When I look at you, I see and feel?"

She nods her head, takes a breath, and pounds some more. "I see an abusive piece of shit touching a little girl when you should have been protecting me, you fucked-up asshole! I feel rage! I feel ashamed! I feel unloved! I feel all alone! Fuck you!"

"And you're angry because?"

"I'm angry because I was a child, you sick piece of shit, and I trusted you and felt safe with you, and you betrayed me, you abusive fucked-up cunt!"

Lisa continues screaming obscenities until she is howling, tears and snot pouring from her eyes and nose.

Mona then says, "And you're sad because?"

Lisa stops hitting the cushion and begins rocking herself gently. "I'm sad because I loved you and trusted you, and you betrayed me."

"And you're mad at you because?"

"I'm mad at me because I felt it was my fault and that I must be bad and unworthy. I lost me in that moment. I'm mad because I rejected me and denied me and abandoned me a long, long time ago."

"And I promise me . . . ?"

"I promise me that I will never lose me again."

"Why?"

"Because I love me and will protect me, all of me, always."

"Why?"

"Because I am beautiful and worthy of love. Because I am a child of God. Because there is a light in me that no one can diminish. Because I am fucking amazing."

I sit there, my heart pressing hard against my chest, wondering if she's talking about her experience or mine? But there's no way she could have known about mine. Still, I feel exposed.

Lisa stands up now, wipes her eyes with the back of her hand, smiles brightly, and says, "Great, thanks, gotta go. Love you, Mona! See you soon! Good luck, Seane! Remember, he didn't fuck you up, you were already fucked up; he's just the catalyst that's going to help you change all that. See ya!"

She bounds out of the room and down the stairs. I hear the animated ghouls sound off as she activates their sensors. I look back at Mona. She smiles, as if all of this were the most normal thing in the world, hands me the racket, and says, "Go ahead, Yogi. Give it a shot!"

I take the racket in my hand. I don't want her to watch me. I don't want to be ugly. *What if I lose control? What if I start hitting the cushion and I can't stop, and I end up smashing the room to bits?* I look down at my trembling hands. Feelings of shame well up in me. *Where's that coming from?* Before I have a chance to consider the answer, feelings of intense rage surface. My face goes hot, my heartbeat quickens. I glance at Mona, who is watching me and waiting. *Fuck her. This is bullshit!* I think, looking quickly away. I want to throw the racket down, get out of this freaky house, and run as far from these feelings as possible. I want to get away from this bizarre woman. But I don't. I look back up at her. Her eyes find mine, and she waits patiently. I realize that I trust her, and I don't know why. I deepen my breath, knowing that the uncomfortable feelings will eventually change. *Breathe and everything . . .*

"Uhhh . . . what are you doing?" Mona asks.

"I'm breathing."

"I get that, but why?"

"It regulates my nervous system. I'm feeling anxious, and that's what I do when I feel anxious."

Mona watches me for a moment, taking me in fully. "Actually," she says quietly, "you are bypassing your emotions when you do that. It's just another skill you've mastered to avoid feeling. It's a good one, better than drugs, but it's still masking your pain. How about just breathing and being fully with the pain at the same time?"

I sit back on the hideous couch and take hold of one of the three stuffed fish nearby. My eyes fill with tears.

"Tell me, what's going on, baby?" she asks.

"I don't want to be with the pain."

"I know, baby. I wish there was an easier way, but to get beyond it, you gotta go through it."

"But my yoga practice teaches me how to be present with uncomfortable sensations. I already do that! I use asana and breathwork to help me ground and discharge the energy. That's what I've been doing for years! And it's worked! Why is it suddenly not enough?"

Mona smiles. "Discharging the energy is good. But perhaps there's something more we can do to help you go deeper. Maybe we can understand what the pain is trying to teach you. Do you believe in God, Seane?"

I nod.

"And you work to be in relationship with God?"

I nod again.

She says, "Well, yoga is about being in connection with everything, right? So, here's the deal. You can't make that connection from your head. Your thoughts, your ego, create separation. You want unity? You find it in your heart. It's never about what you think; it's always about how you feel. Because God is love. It's your vulnerability that will lead you to surrender all that you *think* you know, and surrendering is how we open to God. So asana is great. It gets into the tension. It allows you to be with the repressed emotions. This is just another layer to the work you're already doing. I want to help you understand how that tension got there in the first place, to see the way in which you are addicted to it and how it keeps you stuck *and* safe. The same way your attachments to your story keep you stuck and safe. I want to help you understand your story and the way it lives within you. I want you to own it and feel it—not just admit it or explain it. I want to help you understand how all of it, even your ex, was meant to bring you to God. You want to find out?"

"Yes." I say, nervously tapping the tennis racket against my foot.

"Then, let's rinse this shit."

I get down onto the floor in front of the cushion and, like the young woman from the closet, raise the racket over my head.

"Fuck you, you cheating, lying, motherfucker!" I say, smashing the racket down.

"Nope. He's not why you're here."

"What do you mean?"

Ignoring my question, she instructs me to bring my arms over my head again and then says, "Fuck you, molester."

I freeze. My eyes widen in astonishment. How did she know? I open my mouth to say something, but she just leans forward, and in a kind, loving, and gentle voice, she says, "Say his name, baby."

"But I'm done with all that!"

"Say his name, baby."

With that, I strike the cushion and say his name, without much conviction. I try again, smashing the racket down harder this time. I keep at it, over and over again, until suddenly, from deep inside, a raging, primal scream erupts, for all the neighborhood to hear. Wild, uncontrollable tears come pouring out, bringing with them all the anger and humiliation and grief I have been holding inside for twenty-five years. I beat the living shit out of that cushion.

"Now say fuck you to all the men who harassed you."

"Fuck you!" I scream, realizing only in that moment how deep the fear and rage of abuse and exploitation is within me. I scream, not only for all I've experienced, but for all the women in my family, and in this world, who have suffered because their bodies were sexualized, raped, taunted, judged, harassed, and accosted.

"And you're angry because . . . ?"

"I am angry because . . . !" And I continue to spew forth all the fury, judgment, and hatred I feel. Every time I start to analyze or "see both sides," Mona interrupts. "Stop over-understanding! You're bypassing! Stay on the feelings!" So, I let all the "ugliness" out, feeling liberated with each word I shout.

"And you're crazy because?"

"I'm not crazy! I've never been crazy! My intuition is on fire! Fuck you to all the people who have made me second-guess myself! I am a motherfucking witch!"

"And fuck you because . . . ?

"Huh?" I say, as I stop mid-slam. "Fuck *me*? Why?"

"Just do it."

"Fuck me." I say weakly. "Fuck me for believing them." I hit the pillow again. "Fuck me for all the ways I gave my power away." I begin to pick up steam. "Fuck me for avoiding my big feelings, for pretending everything was okay when it wasn't, and for looking for love from men who were broken themselves." By now I'm pounding away, my hands burning from the friction. "Fuck me for abandoning me! Fuck me! Fuck me!"

Finally, lying on the floor, the energy discharged, sweat dripping down my face, tendrils of hair stuck to my mouth, I feel spent. Mona says quietly, "And I forgive you because . . . ?"

Not taking my eyes off of Mona, I sit up, put down my racquet, and, as though I were channeling something outside of myself, I say, "I forgive you because I must. Because I no longer want to carry you or this story within me. I forgive you because there is a bigger purpose to you being in my life, and I want to understand what you were here to teach me. I forgive you because resentment is an energy that is hurting me and preventing me from feeling me. I forgive you because you are human and broken and have your own deep pain that I can never know or understand. I forgive you because I have no interest in staying stuck in a moment in time that doesn't serve my joy. It was real, and it hurt, but it's only a part of my story. What you did does not define me. It is not who I am. I refuse to remain tethered to your pain, rage, shame, or denial."

Everything pouring out of me was the truth. It was from another level of "knowing." For the first time, I could get a sense of the deep hurt and the fear that must live within the heart of my molester and all the men who have harassed and hurt me. I felt a genuine sense of empathy, not for their choices or their actions, but for the soul within them trying to emerge but unable to because of their own trauma, or karma, or whatever the fuck it is that disconnects any of us from our true nature. It was never personal. It was spiritual. Just like Mona said. Whether or not they "get it" is not my business. It's between them and their own God. My work is to call my power back and to grow and love and learn and open not in spite of my journey, but *because* of it. All of it.

"And your ex?" Mona asks.

"Ugh. Can I hold onto that anger a little longer?"

"Sure, baby! It's all up to you. Just as long as you know where we're going with this."

"I do," I reply. "So, is it done then? Am I healed?"

Mona just laughs. "I doubt it, baby. Ten minutes from now you may get triggered all over again, and you'll fall back into your resentment and blame and rail at the world for how unfair and cruel it is. Remember empowerment is a process. But for this moment, you have glimpsed what is possible. You got a taste of what it means to call your power back. This is how you develop your self-confidence. Self-confidence comes from knowing who you really are—in here." She points to my heart and taps it. "When you know that, you will always be whole. By rinsing the crazy voices, by releasing the animal rage, you give voice to the ego and let the shadow self out. This creates space for the truth hidden under the suppression to make its way to the surface. You have always known the truth, baby, because God is here." She taps on my chest again. "And God speaks to you from here." She gently thumps my third eye. "It's in your intuition. You know what intuition means? It's in-tuition. Inner teaching. It lives within you. The shadow just blocks the light. Just keep doing your work. Do your yoga, keep grounding and moving that energy. Just don't bypass any emotion. Feel it all! Be in relationship with it and let it liberate your true nature. Isn't that what yoga is? Look to the root of your suffering. Be with it, rinse it, and then flip the story. See who your teachers are and the way they are leading you to love."

I think of the bee.

Mona continues. "Doing the work will give you insight into why you are here on this planet, what you are supposed to learn, and how it will lead to your purpose. But all of that is for another day. Today you got a glimpse into the truth. That's enough."

"What do you mean, my purpose?"

"Oh sweetie," she says. "Sometimes our pain is our purpose. And the very thing you have been running from, once empowered, becomes the very place from which you will serve. It's the gift of karma. It's called empathy," she leans forward and whispers in my ear, "and it's what will heal this world."

TEACHINGS FROM THE PAIN
HEALING, FORGIVENESS, AND OWNING THE TRUTH

No words could ever adequately describe the whirlwind of brilliance, beauty, and fabulousness that was Mona Miller. I say "was" because in July 2011, weeks after her fiftieth birthday and eleven months after my dad died, Mona was killed in a tragic car accident. She left behind her child, her partner Bernadette, and a vast wealth of teachings that live on in the hearts of her many students, mine included.

It's impossible to break down all that Mona taught me about how to see, feel, and embrace every part of myself and how to engage in the world in a compassionate and powerful way. But I will give it my best shot because what Mona taught *was* yoga, although I doubt she'd call it that. It was about being in relationship with all aspects of yourself—the light and the shadow—making peace with them and allowing them to teach you about your humanity, about the power of your ever-expanding consciousness, and about the importance of forgiveness, gratitude, and seeing the Divine in

all. The best part? With her over-the-top personality and her willingness to see beauty everywhere, she brought a lightness of being to everything she did—she reminded me to laugh often, love big, and find meaning even in the incomprehensible.

Make no mistake though. No matter how many candy corns she put in her candy dish or how many show tunes she belted out on her white baby grand, nothing Mona ever did was easy. The pathway was raw, intimate, and honest; it required breaking shame, being relentlessly self-aware, feeling big emotions—no intellectualizing or bypassing allowed—and pushing through resistance to uncover the beauty of our true Self. Mona, like Billy, believed that *everything* is Spirit and all experiences are spiritual—even (and sometimes, especially) the ones we think are messed-up. Every moment can open us to our divine potential and, in fact, what gets in our way *is the way.*

Mona helped me understand what happens when we get caught up in our egos and become attached to the illusions (the stories) we hold onto and tell ourselves are true. Yoga showed me where my stories live. Mona taught me how to give voice to them, embrace them fully, and then give them back to God. Yoga gave my narrative a presence; Mona gave it expression. The two practices together empowered me to find my voice and to see purpose and beauty in every moment—the good and the bad, the light and the shadow—as flip sides to the same coin that leads to transcendence.

SPIRIT AND SOUL

Mona's work was steeped in Spirit; she framed all experience through the lens of Grace. She lived by the saying, "We are spiritual beings having a human experience." But what does that mean? It means that we are more than the sum total of our experiences in this body, more than the stories we tell ourselves, and more than the stories we hide from ourselves. We are Spirit. And Spirit is the direct manifestation of Source, or God, what the ancient yoga texts refer to as Universal Consciousness or *purusha*. It is primordial, the "breath within the breath," as Rumi once said—perfect, pure, eternal, and unchangeable.

The soul is our individual expression of Spirit; it is also immune to birth and death and never loses its individuality. The soul is what makes me "me" and you "you," the "I AM" essence in each of us. It's connected to (but not affected by) our emotions, physical sensations, impulses, and desires. Without the soul, the body has no awareness; without the soul, we cannot express ourselves. Some say that the seat of the soul resides in the heart (in the anahata chakra) and is what awakens within us an inherent capacity for compassion, connection, and love. Spirit, they say, resides at the crown (in the sahasrara chakra) and awakens us to Source, to our divinity. In truth, there is no separation between soul and Spirit—the former is simply the individual expression of the latter.

The soul's work is to remember; the Spirit's work is to be. The soul is invested in this remembering, this knowing, but doesn't identify with it. It wants to understand the shadow because it's only through human experience that consciousness can evolve. It wants experience, welcomes it, and draws it inward. The soul bears witness to our humanity—without getting sucked in or attached—and awakens from it.

Our ego or "small self" is busy having a different reality, however. Our ego latches onto whatever is in front of it and won't let go, believing that what it sees or experiences is real life, permanent and unchanging. The ego constantly reminds us that we are separate from others, from the planet, and from God. This ultimately leads to suffering because, of course, nothing is permanent, and there is no separation. We suffer when we believe that our fear, doubt, anxiety, or heartbreak is real and forever, that we'll never be happy, healthy, financially successful, or in love again. We also suffer when we become attached to pleasure, when we believe that our happiness, love, health, and financial success is permanent—because it isn't! Either way, defining ourselves by external validation or material worth is a tried-and-true recipe for misery.

Even if it aches with pain, the ego doesn't want to change because change is frightening; it represents the unknown, that which can't be controlled. So, it remains steadfastly attached to what it believes to be true, in order to survive. It clings to its judgments—this is good, that is bad; this is right, that is wrong—in order to distinguish itself from the perceived "other," to give itself meaning and purpose. The soul, on the other hand, says, "Experience? Hell, yeah. Bring it on." The soul wants experience so it can know itself in relation to the ego, to the shadow.

What Mona drilled into my head was that light cannot exist without dark. To understand and truly embrace the illuminated Self or Spirit, we have to understand and embrace the wisdom of the ego and the shadow. The shadow is also our teacher, and we must learn how to be in relationship with it and listen to what it has to teach us about our humanity, otherwise it will dictate the choices we make and the way we experience the world.

Everything is connected. There is no separation, no matter how hard the ego tries. To know acceptance, we must also experience rejection. To know patience, we must also know resistance; to know understanding, we must also know judgment; to know love, we must also understand fear and respect its power. We cannot learn to forgive without first feeling betrayed. And we cannot bypass the tremors of life, its heartbreaks and its losses, because without those, we will never fully know joy. The soul requires all of this in order to grow and heal; the soul draws in exactly what our consciousness needs for that growth to happen.

This is what it means to be fully human. We must live it all. We must take life in and witness our response. Once we see where we resist and what we react to, we can begin to uncover who we are—our authentic nature, our highest Self—and who we are to each other. When we enter into a relationship with Spirit, we develop real Self-confidence—with a capital *S*—and we begin to see who we are beyond our ego and understand why we're here and what we need to accomplish. As a result of that, we can embrace the totality of our authentic nature and trust our intuition, or what I call the inner teachings of God. This is the crux of Mona's work and, in a very real way, of yoga. It's a far cry from the ego's version of self-confidence, which the ego attaches to aspects of being that are ephemeral, such as beauty, money, power, and fame. What happens when the beauty fades, the money dries up,

and the power and fame evaporate? All that is left is emptiness until we're able to refill the confidence tank with another external validation.

FLIPPING THE STORY

Much of Mona's work was about seeing the limitations of our perceptions, recognizing where and why we give away power, and learning how to call it back. We retrieve our lost power, she said, when we understand the spiritual necessity and significance of each and every event in our life, even the fucked-up ones, when we recognize that everything that happens is an opportunity for spiritual growth. This process of self-understanding is not an intellectual one; it's primal.

I have to admit I didn't want to see my ex's betrayal as a spiritual opportunity. It sucked. He broke my heart. I was devastated. Mona told me not to worry. I would come to understand why he was in my life and why I was in his, but not right away. First, she said, I needed to override my rational thinking mind (the manomaya kosha) and engage the emotional body (the pranamaya kosha) through a process she called "rinsing." Rinsing included yelling, screaming, or hitting a pillow with a racket—often all three at once—anything that would physically and emotionally discharge energy. Once that discharge happened, the stuck emotion had space to free itself, express itself, and move up and out of the body and the subconscious. I had experienced some of that in Bryan's class, and through trauma work, so it wasn't completely foreign to me. But Mona didn't stop there. She then guided me to "process," which meant diving deeper into my trauma and mental-emotional attachments (what she called our personal narratives), peeling away the layers of ego and illusion, until I could "flip the story."

Flipping the story means reinterpreting an event from a larger spiritual perspective and understanding its divine purpose beyond how the small self perceives it. Through a process of self-reflection, rinsing, and radical accountability—without bypassing the teachings of the shadow self—we can begin to heal our own pain body, as well as develop empathy for the fragile humanity of *all* the people involved in our story, without judgment, *especially* those who have caused us pain. This process requires us to understand the ways we "co-create" with Spirit to manifest what is essential for our soul's growth, to see the brutal and crucial role of forgiveness for personal healing, to willingly "own" how each experience is in service to our awakening, and to recognize its role in our soul's evolution toward Oneness. Oh, and, while we're at it, to cultivate gratitude for each experience as it is without wishing that it could be or should be different. That's a lot! But, that was Mona.

The easiest way to explain Mona's work is through the yogic lens of karma. Karma means "action" and suggests that everything we do in the present will eventually affect us in the future. Everything we did in the past informs our present reality. Our actions create our destiny, and the results of those actions influence who we are and who we will become. Life doesn't happen *to* us; it happens *for* us, and it is the cause and effect of all our past karmas. In other words, karma reflects back to us where we have not made skillful, conscious choices and gives us the opportunity to try again, to heal any suffering we've caused others or ourselves. If we don't get it the first time, or the hundredth time, that experience will keep manifesting over and over again (often in different guises) until we do. It is through karma that we learn to heed our wisdom mind and act with compassion and empathy. When Mona insisted that I name the one who harmed me, she wasn't talking about my ex. She was talking about the man who had molested me when I was a child. Until I could say his name, until I could see him, feel the pain of my young self, and express my anger, humiliation, and helplessness, I would continue to enter into relationships that were lopsided, in which I gave my power away, in which I had no voice.

As Mona used to tell me, "Everything happens exactly the way it's supposed to for the soul to transform." But that doesn't mean what happened was preordained. It just means shit happens. And, when it does, there's no changing it. It's just life. You can assign meaning to it, absolutely. You can heal and become wiser, more empowered, and more empathetic—not in spite of the circumstance or event, but because of it.

COMMITTING TO THE WORK

The work I did with Mona was, in some ways, the hardest thing I've ever done in my life. It took discipline and a fierce determination I didn't even know I had to keep showing up. This relentless dedication to the work, the commitment to take charge of our own destiny, is what yoga calls tapas. It's not the first time I practiced tapas, of course. I relied on it to keep me from climbing back up when I sat in the stairwell of my East Village apartment building, willing myself not to revert to my old OCD patterning. It's what gave me the willpower and the singleness of purpose I needed in India to trust my instincts. But Mona took it to a whole new level. With her, I dedicated myself—over and over again—to the process of discovering the truth, regardless of where it might lead me. The Yoga Sutras say that the practice you should embrace is one that will help you gain inner stability, introduce you to yourself, and allow you to see the unfiltered truth. I don't recommend doing such intense work without a competent teacher supporting you, however. I know I couldn't have done any of it without Mona's fierce and skillful guidance.

Introducing you to yourself means remembering and embodying everything that makes you you, including the cringeworthy or traumatic experiences you've hidden away or "forgotten." It means learning to trust your intuition. To do that requires a strong and steady foundation. You must feel rooted and connected both to the earth and to a force beyond that. Your inner wisdom will open you up to the flow of life, unencumbered by the illusions that keep you tethered to your smaller mind. A regular asana practice grounds the body, and chakra work exposes the emotional fissures that influence your ability to stay steady and present. Only when we are stable, are we free to fly.

Early in my relationship with Mona, she told me to prepare myself for what awakening might look like. "It will require you to confront anything that is blocking you from your highest potential," she said. "Once you set your intention and open yourself to healing, you will also invite in that which scares you the most and keeps you from your highest Self. It's not because you're being punished—quite the opposite. It's because that which scares you is also what keeps you from the truth of your soul. In confronting what you resist and the fears that come with that resistance, you discover the gold within

the resistance itself. It is alchemy of the spirit. That is the journey toward wholeness." That is tapas.

FEELING INTO THE PAIN

Once we commit to the work, we must move full-on into svadhyaya, the yogic path of self-awareness and self-reflection. Once again, this was a familiar path for me. Over the years my yoga practice has showed me—sometimes gently, other times pretty forcefully—what I had been incapable of seeing, or, let's get real, what I refused to see. Svadhyaya is the *soul's work*, the soul's investigation into how things are. It invites us to look at experience as experience—without labeling it. It's about becoming intimately familiar with what our ego has to teach us—without judging or locking anything away—so there are no surprises. We need to see, listen, and feel all of it so the soul can learn what the shadow self has to teach, and so we can eventually uncover the Divine presence at the core of our being—under all the fog, confusion, and doubt, and all the shame and blame we pile on. It's not about *understanding* your pain, as Mona said to me, or even articulating it, which, by the way, I excelled at. It's about *feeling* it, which I sucked at.

Before I met Mona, I was a master at describing how I felt (admitting my feelings) without actually having to feel anything. I could use spiritual language to rise above the messiness of my "baser" self. Mona didn't allow me to bypass the shadow self—and she'd call me on it every time. We must be willing to "go get it," she said, own it, and be in full relationship with it. Go beyond the admitting, beyond the noticing—which was all ego-driven—and name our feelings, *feel* them, get down into the muck, and engage with them. She insisted that I confront my feelings, rail against them, and mourn all that I felt I had lost. In Mona's words, I needed to rinse this shit out of me. Rinsing makes space for total self-acceptance and joyous self-reunion. It insists, in the words of Nikki Myers, my friend and yoga teacher extraordinaire, that we acknowledge the "Fuck you" before we can get to the "Bless you."

In order to get the shit out of us, we must let our crazy voices speak, Mona used to say. If we don't give them permission to come forward and say what they need to say, they'll just keep getting louder and louder. We will never learn what they have to teach us, nor will we ever be able to set them free. They will always cloud our thinking and separate us from the truth.

Release came that day in Bryan's class as a lifetime of tears poured out of me, carrying with them the anger, anxiety, fear, and grief buried deep in my cells. I welcomed the little girl, whom I had abandoned so long ago, back into my awareness. But it wasn't until I worked with Mona that I allowed my young, beautiful self to speak for herself—unfiltered. Only then could I feel the rage, humiliation, and shame that continued to live inside of me all those years after my molestation. Only then could I begin to understand what my pain was trying to teach me. Only then could I release it.

The practice of svadhyaya doesn't always have to be a big cathartic event; in fact, it shouldn't be. Don't feel like you have to dredge up *all* that you are, all at once, all the time. Svadhyaya is about noticing and then reflecting on what you notice. It's not really a prescription for change; it's an invitation to discover who you already are so you can move forward with confidence and clarity. Becoming self-aware allows you to enter into a relationship with your past, but it also encourages you to be fully present to your interactions and reactions, *as they are happening.* There may be times in which what begins to surface proves to be too much to handle. That's okay too. Acknowledge what's coming up, bring it to light, and ask it for more time.

GETTING TO THE BLESS YOU

Of course, tapas and svadhyaya are what we need in order for the soul to evolve, for healing to begin. Tapas keeps us showing up; svadhyaya shines a light on the shadow so we can see what we've refused to see and be in relationship with *every* experience, *every* person in our lives. Ishvara pranidhana asks us to strip away the judgments we've held onto and stand naked in the mystery. Ishvara pranidhana also means radical openness; it is what puts the brakes on the ego, stops us in our tracks, and

brings us back to God. The sting of the bee in Pondicherry; the sound of the gong in Gurmukh's class that landed me in my body and showed me all that is beautiful, powerful, tender, and whole; and, of course, Billy's insistence that God was in Danny, and Violet, and everyone else in Heaven.

When we surrender the hold the ego's small-minded agenda has on us and embrace the truth, we can move, think, and interact more from our heart (the wisdom mind). We let go of the false belief that we are somehow separate from others, that we deserve love and understanding, while those who have harmed us deserve to be punished and shunned. It's not about bypassing circumstances we don't like or getting rid of people we find deeply irritating. It's about letting go of anything that stands in our way of forgiving and, ultimately, serving.

Tapas, svadhyaya, and ishvara pranidhana formed a framework for Mona's work. She insisted we show up completely (tapas) and notice what blocks our path to the Divine (svadhyaya). And then, rinse that shit out of us—the ego and all the crazy voices—so that we could get to the truth (ishvara pranidhana). The only way to get to the truth, to illuminate the soul, Mona said, was to feel everything and walk side-by-side with our own humanity.

Once we can do that, we can begin to forgive. I got a taste of that back at YogaWorks, when Bryan asked everyone in class to forgive themselves. That was the first step in calling my power back. The second step was to forgive those who had harmed me—that was harder. And finally, I had to really *see* them, *feel* their suffering, and let go of the idea that my suffering was somehow more wretched and more justified than theirs. *That* was the hardest of all.

FORGIVENESS

Forgiveness is absolutely imperative for healing to happen. But it can't happen unless we do the work, accept the whole of our being fully in love, and then break down the barriers that separate us from the "other."

We are all here to awaken, to evolve our soul, but we can't do that as long as we're immune to the suffering of others. We all have trauma—our own and what we've inherited from our ancestors; we all have stuff to work out in the unconscious; we all have conditioning, belief systems, and bullshit we've acquired over a lifetime of experiences. We're all learning, growing, and trying to remember the essential light, and love, of our own being-ness. But here's the thing. We can't expand our own consciousness and forgive ourselves for our human frailties and then turn around and judge someone else as being broken or flawed when they're just working out their shit too.

To forgive is probably the toughest spiritual practice we will face in life. But forgive we must in order to release the caustic energy festering within us, making us sick, and separating us from our highest Self—and from each other. Forgive because we recognize that we are all flawed, all broken to some degree, all traumatized, all human. Ignore the story and see the soul. The people who have hurt us may be assholes, but they are also children of God, like we all are. So give them back to God. Pray they learn, heal, and open to love. It is this forgiveness that unites, and it is this forgiveness that heals. And just when you think you've fully forgiven, forgive again. This process takes time, but it's worth it; in the end, you get your Self back. Fully and whole.

I could not be free until I forgave my ex-boyfriend. I could not transcend suffering until I forgave my molester and every other harasser, manipulator, and abuser. Forgiving them never once meant that I condoned their behavior. Not even a little bit. Forgiveness means I refuse to carry them, their energy, their wounds, and their story within me. As long as I stay stuck in the story, bound to them in negativity, I can never break free. Our commingled pain will continue to influence my present and my future choices and keep me disconnected from my truth.

Forgiveness is much more than understanding or wishing someone well. It's essential for our own liberation. Before I could forgive my ex, I needed to see him as flawed. He was an asshole—he's the one who broke my heart—and I was a victim. I could rinse my anger, hurt, and sadness, but that wasn't enough. I had to understand that none of what went down was personal. It was spiritual. Then, I needed to see it all from that spiritual perspective so I could understand its divine purpose. I needed to figure out who we were to

each other and how we contributed to one another's spiritual growth. Otherwise, karmically, I would continue to magnetize more lovers and partners like him in my life, again and again, until I finally learned the lessons necessary to understand that I am not a victim, I am a child of God, and I'm on a path to learn the power of love. Equally important and yet so hard to admit: so is he.

On a spiritual level, my ex and I were exactly where we needed to be for our individual souls to evolve. Although I would much rather have learned my lesson in an easier way, he was my teacher, and I was his. It made sense. I craved intimacy and feared it at the same time. I had a hard time letting go of people in my life (even when I knew I should) and had issues of abandonment. These were the things that separated me from God. So, whom did I choose? Someone whose fear of intimacy was as complex as mine and who checked out the moment things got either too comfortable or too complicated. Someone who feared rejection so much that he skipped out before he could be left behind. These were the things that separated him from God. The unconscious was playing itself out in both of us. To heal ourselves, our shadows needed excavation. We were each other's mirror, and we were absolutely 100 percent perfect for each other. At least our shadow selves thought so.

Reframing the story this way helped me see how my ex and I had come together—and fallen apart—at just the right time to learn what we both needed to learn. At that moment, I stopped being a victim. I also stopped abandoning myself and learned the importance of having an intimate connection with myself before looking for that in someone else. What about my ex? Did he manage to "get it" too? It doesn't matter. It's actually none of my business. That's between him and the God of his own understanding. True liberation came when I could see the wounds he carried, underneath all his unconscious and hurtful behavior, and honor the tenderness, and true beauty, of his soul.

Don't for a moment think that this is spiritual bypass or a Pollyanna moment. It's pretty impossible to go down the forgiveness road without doing some serious self-reflection first, to find the "Bless you" without acknowledging the "Fuck you." I needed to give voice to

my pain, rinse it from my cells, before I could see the humanity in the man who had broken my heart—in spite of his hurtful behavior. I had to surrender my victimhood in order to discover the ways in which our relationship was in service to our souls' evolution, the ways in which it uncovered the truth.

And what is this truth? The truth is that we are here to awaken to the light, to the God within us and within all. How do we do that? By experiencing all of life, without creating separation. By healing the fractured parts of ourselves and accepting the gifts every one of our relationships has to give. By seeing the soul of every being as a pure expression of that person's own divinity. Finally, by letting ourselves love the whole messy, chaotic, *and* beautiful process of "being" that can bring us home to the God within.

All the yoga classes I had taken, all the meditating I had done, and all the deep inner work I had committed to helped prepare me for Mona. Somehow, her wild wisdom and unconventional ways helped me look honestly at my inner life, break the shame I had, share without holding back, and process the shit out of the fear, rage, humiliation, and grief that the little girl in me had carried for so long. The way I teach, the prayers I speak, and the words I write—especially in this book—are all expressions of that work and reflections of the time I spent flipping the narrative from one of blame, victimization, and resentment to one of compassion, empowerment, and gratitude. The reason I can be honest, authentic, raw, and open about my experiences today is because they do not define me. They are simply aspects of my journey, vital for the evolution of my soul and for "remembering" who I truly am beyond my body and my limited thoughts. Just like Billy said. Our life, with all the experiences that come with it, doesn't always look the way we think it should, but that doesn't mean there isn't purposefulness in every moment. Blame and resentments are energies that deplete our physical and emotional bodies—natural impulses derived from our ego self—but they are not who we are. Love is who we are; love is our true nature. The energy of forgiveness refills our reserves and allows us to be fully expressed in the Self. Forgiveness unites, resentment separates. As long as we remain in separation on a personal level, we are perpetuating the very disconnect we wish to transform on a global one. The work begins within us: we must uncover the love we are. And then, as yoga teaches, we must give it away. We are obligated to share it with the world, and when we do, we will come to know, over and over again, the power of that love to awaken the soul to its deepest purpose. And that purpose? To lead a revolution from within for the benefit of all—in the name of equality, justice, freedom, and, of course, love.

And lead we must. Because lives are at stake; freedom, equality, and liberty are at stake. The revolution that will heal this world begins NOW, and your participation is essential. So, what do you say? Are you ready to be a force for change? From the inside out? From love? If your answer is yes, then buckle up . . .

PART II

REVOLUTION OF THE SOUL

In order to see, you have to stop
being in the middle of the picture.

SRI AUROBINDO

ANSWERING THE CALL

9

I HAVE A PHOTO of myself taken around 1990 at a pro-choice rally in New York's Union Square. I'm standing on a riser, holding a megaphone in one hand with the opening pressed to my mouth. My other arm is raised to the sky. The picture cuts off at my wrist, so I can't tell if my hand is clenched in a fist or if my third finger is raised in a fuck-you, but I know it must be one of the two. Just below me is a group of so-called pro-life activists, holding pictures of dead and mutilated babies, clutching Bibles, and waving homemade signs that say "BABY KILLER" and "GOD HATES ABORTION." We have our own paraphernalia we're waving in their faces in defiant response. If you look closely though, all the people in the picture, myself included, have their mouths wide open, screaming something, and their eyes tightly shut.

Everyone was speaking, no one was listening, and no one could see who or what was in front of them. With eyes closed, fists clenched, and mouths opened, we had contracted around our own ideas, shut out our opposition, and blocked the pathway that could have led to dialogue or at least a sliver of understanding. This picture speaks a thousand words. Although I am a strong believer in protesting—it is what makes a democracy truly great—it can also be ineffective when practiced unskillfully.

The picture reflected that perfectly and shows how awful I was as an activist, how inadequate my understanding of service was, and how the tactics (on both sides) weren't exactly conducive to changing hearts or minds. Needless to say, it didn't take long before I burned out.

By the time I landed in LA, I seriously needed a break from all the protests and marches that had defined my activism for so long. And anyway, by 1999, I was working full time, busting my ass as a yoga teacher, teaching at YogaWorks twelve times a week and doing at least as many private sessions. My days were full, and I was very happy. I loved teaching and felt so honored to share a practice that had had such a positive impact on my life. Each day, I would drive from the studio in Santa Monica to various homes in Malibu, Brentwood, or Hollywood and back again. I hustled hard and didn't have much time for anything other than work and my own personal practice.

Something was missing though. Living on the west side of LA, most of the people I was teaching had the access and resources to afford whatever they wanted, including yoga. Obviously I was very grateful for the abundance coming my way, but I also knew that all abundance—financial, physical, emotional, and spiritual—was energy, and that energy had to keep flowing outward. If not, it would get stuck and stagnate. I certainly didn't want the run of opportunities and good luck I'd been enjoying to come to a screeching halt. I knew I needed to reciprocate in some way, but how?

I decided to ask Mona.

When I brought it up at our next session, Mona said, "Just be of service, oh Holy One." But I did nothing. I brought it up again at our session after that. She looked at me and said, "Uh . . . I have an idea. Try service." Still I did nothing. I brought it up one more time. She just shook her head and rolled her eyes. Much later, after running around doing errands, I noticed a sticky note that had fallen off the back of my sweater. It said: "BE OF SERVICE TO THE WORLD!" Got it. I need to give back and serve my community in a way that benefits others, not just my wallet. Problem was, I had no idea how best to *do* that. I knew that I didn't want to jump back into frontline activism, staging protests and railing against injustice. I still felt pretty burned-out. My outrage was real, of course, and my commitment strong, but my participation was less than stellar.

So, yes, I was eager to serve—but doing what? The only real skill I had was teaching yoga. Then I should teach yoga. But, to whom? I liked teenagers, and I was pretty sure I could help them. I did a little research, looking into the juvenile detention centers in LA—not many yoga programs there. Unfortunately, it was almost impossible to get through the interview process. As soon as they heard "yoga," they'd answer, "No, thank you." Apparently, touching those in lock-up was frowned upon.

▼

Then one day I see a feature on the local news about a shelter in the Los Angeles area, which housed, educated, and provided health care and psychological support for young people between the ages of eleven and seventeen who have been arrested and put through the system for being adolescent prostitutes.

I can't stand that phrase, "adolescent prostitutes," which is used to describe teens whose bodies are sold for sex. These young people have been severely and unimaginably sexually abused and often trafficked—sometimes by their own families. They are seriously victimized and, to me, the term "adolescent prostitute" sounds as though they were complicit in the choice to sell their bodies. These children have been manipulated and used by their pimps or families, introduced to drugs and alcohol, joined gangs, and run through the system, including jail. They have been betrayed, abandoned, and as you can imagine, highly traumatized, often by the very people and systems meant to protect them.

I immediately know I need to work with these kids. I can't get them out of my head. I'm horrified by the unimaginable trauma they've experienced and grateful that a facility exists to help them heal. Yoga would be so great for them; I just knew it. So I reach out and set up a meeting with the director of the shelter. When I arrive, she orders a background check and then asks me why I've come and what I envision doing there. I tell her about the benefits of yoga for healing the body, mind, and spirit, how it helps with stress and focus, and how it could support these youths to feel better in their bodies and improve their digestion, habits, and overall health and wellness. She listens, asks a few questions, and then ushers me out the door.

A month and two more interviews later, she calls to let me know that I've been approved. And then she lays down the rules: I can't talk about sex, love, their families, or their pimps. I'm not allowed to ask them about their time on the streets or why many of them are wearing "engagement" rings. I can't touch them, and they can't touch each other. They can't do any movement or posture that might be sensual or sexually explicit. I can't say "healing," "trauma," "acceptance," or "forgiveness." I can't say "God" or "Spirit" or pray in any way. I can't use any word that might make them angry, upset, scared, or triggered. I can't ask about their tattoos or the scars on their bodies, especially the ones that appear self-inflicted. I can't talk about myself.

I bob my head enthusiastically. "Absolutely. No problem. Totally get it. Can't wait!" I hang up the phone. What the hell have I just signed up for?

The shelter is housed in a nondescript, large cement building surrounded by gates and security cameras. I'm buzzed in, surrender my ID, and follow the receptionist through a hallway of offices and bedrooms. It's a Tuesday evening, and the children have just eaten dinner. Doing yoga after a meal isn't ideal, but it's the only time they can spare. The rest of their day is devoted to regular school classes, individual and group therapy, life skills, and meetings with legal counsel.

As I glance into the small, neat rooms, I see pictures of movie, rock, and rap stars hanging on the walls, interspersed with handmade drawings of hearts, animals, and inspirational quotes. I notice all kinds of stuffed animals on the beds, which are covered in shades of pink, purple, blue, and yellow. The sense of normalcy feels like a disconnect, but I remind myself that these are children, severely abused children perhaps, but children nonetheless. Why shouldn't their rooms look like most teenagers' rooms? The director brings me into a common room to meet the fifteen young people who are living there. There are thirteen girls and two boys, one of whom is transgender, and I notice that no one is white except the two counselors and me.

The kids lounge around lazily, watching TV and chatting. The counselors rally them to get ready for class. Glancing up from the couches they're sprawled across, they give me a once-over. I look down at my black Danskin leggings and tight tank top with "Om Girl" written across it and wonder what they think of me. They roll their eyes, smirk, and turn their attention back to the TV, and I have their answer. I regret my tank top choice immediately. The counselors tell them again, a little more firmly, to get up. One by one they amble over to where I've laid out the mats, and flop down. They could not be less interested.

I smile and nervously introduce myself. One girl whispers, "Cornhole," under her breath when she hears my last name; the other kids crack up. I laugh uncomfortably and glance over at the counselors. They frown, but gesture for me to continue. I start to explain the benefits of yoga but keep tripping over my words, feeling awkward and self-conscious, afraid I'll say something stupid. Shit. I'm intimidated. By a bunch of fourteen-year-olds? What the hell? Now I'm really anxious.

I invite them to sit up and attempt to bring them into meditation. "Sitting tall," I say, using my most soothing yoga voice, "and feeling your buttocks . . ." *Buttocks?* They fall over laughing, grabbing suggestively at their bottoms. I look at the counselors again. They just shake their heads. I take a different route and ask them to close their eyes, but they refuse, no matter how many times I ask. So, I try another tactic and say, "Keeping your spine tall and straight, imagine there's a string attached to your head and someone is pulling you upward by the string, lifting you toward the ceiling." This cracks them up even more and some start acting like they are puppets with strings that move them. Crap. I try again to ground them, the tone of my voice a bit sterner this time, but they are now poking at each other, or staring off into space, or picking at their toenails. This clearly is not going well.

I've never worked with young people before—and certainly not those with serious trauma. I just want to tell them to knock it the fuck off and pay attention, but I don't know how to do that without coming off as aggressive and potentially causing harm. I want them to like me, but I also want them to do as I say. I keep looking over at the counselors, but they're now chatting with each other and ignoring us. I am in way over my head.

For the next hour, I attempt to teach yoga, but the kids are absolutely horrible. They make fun of me, fart and snap each other's bra straps, and anything else they can think of to insult me. Every once in a while, the counselors come to my rescue and tell them to pay attention, not touch each other, or be respectful. I do everything I can to engage them and get them to try the poses, but the more I instruct, the more disruptive, rude, and bored they become. The whole hour is a complete mess; they know it and take great delight in my discomfort. I watch the clock and can't wait for this fiasco to end so I can leave. I'm sure they feel the same way.

When the hour is up, I roll up my mat, thank them, and manage a feeble good-bye. The girl who called me Cornhole flips me the finger. Another one makes a blow-job gesture, pumping her closed fist toward her mouth and pushing her tongue into the inside of her cheek. The other kids think that's hysterical, and the room explodes with laughter. The last thing I hear, as I leave the room, is a counselor telling them to cut it out. I nearly run past their bedrooms with the stuffed animals and hearts on the wall. I stand impatiently at the reception desk, waiting for my ID and to be buzzed out so I can get as far away from this fucking place as possible.

Once outside I see creepy-looking men lurking around the gates. The security guard tells them to beat it and explains to me that they're pimps trying to make contact with "their" kids. I move quickly toward my car, and as I do, I notice the pimps edging back toward the perimeter of the property. My body feels hot, my legs weak and trembling; I need to sit down. I make it to the front seat, and suddenly I am flooded with emotion. Rage erupts from the depths of my being. I breathe. I think of Mona, and I know she'd encourage me to give voice to my anger.

"Fuck them!" I scream and immediately feel guilty. They're just kids; they've been through so much. Why am I being so judgmental? Where's my compassion? *Don't bypass, Seane. Rinse the crazy voices! Let the "judger" speak!* Okay, okay, here goes . . .

"Fuck those mean, little assholes! They don't stand a chance in this world. There's no way they will get the help they need. I mean, who's going to want to help them? Besides, they don't even know they *need* help. They're just angry and pathetic and used up and fucked up, and nothing can change that!"

Wow. That's what I'm feeling? That's what's in my body? Damn. Where did this come from? *Stop analyzing and start rinsing! Go deeper, Seane. Let the "martyr" speak!*

"Don't they know help when they see it? Ungrateful little bitches. What the fuck? I came all this way to teach them, and they treat me like shit? What about *my* needs? I'm an experienced yoga teacher! This is the mother fuckin' thanks I get?"

I watch my shaking hands for a moment. I don't like this. "The system is bullshit. Fuck the system! These kids will end up back on the street, addicted to drugs, pregnant before sixteen, pumping out more drug-addicted babies . . . that somehow

I will have to pay for! Why should I be responsible? I have my own issues!" This rant continues—the anger, ignorance, bias, prejudice, and judgment cascading through my whole system. I don't try to stop or even understand any of it. I just let the tears flow. *Get to the truth underneath it, Seane.*

"FUCK!" I scream, over and over, hitting my hands on the steering wheel as I do. Then I stop, my heart still pounding, and stare out onto the street in front of me.

Son of a bitch, I think. That goddamn bee is back.

I turn my attention to the sensations in my body: I breathe, but the breath feels jagged and impatient. I don't want to explore what's underneath, but I know I must. Something's been revealed to me that could hold the key to my growth. But what?

I look out my window. I see one of the pimps sitting on the curbside nearby, smoking a cigarette, and staring intently at the shelter. I know what I need to do. I reach into the glove compartment, grab some scrap paper and a pen, and begin to write, "Dear children, when I look at you, I see . . . When I look at you, I feel . . ."

The next day I visit Mona and tell her that I just met fifteen living, breathing reflections of my suppressed shadow self . . . and they scared the living shit out of me.

Mona laughs and says, "Of course you did, baby. What did you expect? You invited them in, and I bet they are mean and wild. Serves you right." She smiles brightly, looking mightily pleased with herself, and then continues. "So . . . Enlightened One, tell me what you saw."

"I saw their rage and their anger, that's for sure." I say. "But I also saw their fear. I watched all the ways they were acting out—all behaviors I've seen in myself. Mona, I couldn't stand it. I didn't know what to do. I wanted out. I wanted to run away."

"When else has that happened, baby?"

"Are you kidding? I bail whenever I'm confronted with shit in others that scares me, especially when it's shit I can't stand in myself, or . . . I sleep with it!" I laugh. Mona laughs too, high-fives me for my self-deprecating self-awareness, and then encourages me to keep going.

"Man," I say, shaking my head, "I judged those kids so harshly. They scared me, and they knew it. I resented them, Mona, even though I knew their behavior wasn't their fault."

"So what are they here to teach you? What did you learn?"

"What did I learn? I learned that I have a lot to learn. That I am still deeply uncomfortable with rage and anger and have a ton of judgment around it. And, damn, I suck at teaching kids!"

"So who *are* these kids to you?"

"I feel like, in some ways, they're a reflection of me—only magnified. They are my disowned self. The parts of me I'm afraid of, the parts I'm ashamed of, the parts of me I judge," I say. "Otherwise I wouldn't have attracted these particular children to me."

"Attracted *to* you?" Mona says. "Don't be so passive. You actively sought those kids out. *You* did this. This is no accident, you working with sexually abused children. It's karma, my love. You created this opportunity for your spiritual growth. Obviously you weren't aware you were doing this, but your unconscious knows exactly what's needed for real healing and awakening to occur. Remember, you can't change it until you see it. Until you discover the ways you are the same . . . *and different.* That part's essential. Those kids are holding up a mirror, and you're only getting a glimpse into the insight they're providing. Just wait. This is spiritual, and they are a gift."

I nod my head in agreement, then say, only half-kidding, "But they're such assholes."

Mona laughs again and says, "Perfect. So are you. The biggest one of all. You'll all get along just fine. Give it time. All the work you've done up to this point has brought you to this moment, and you are more than ready to see the bigger picture, to understand why things have happened the way they have. Your pain is your purpose and . . ."

"What does that even mean? You've said it before."

Taking a swig from her ever-present 32-ounce Coke, she says, "Guru, go home and process what you've experienced. Let those big feelings out. Don't suppress anything. Do some yoga to release the tension, do your breathing exercises to stay grounded, do your anger work, write out all the big feelings that come up without any judgment—and then pray for those kids."

"Pray for them?" This was a new assignment. "How?"

With that, Mona picks up her Blackberry and, ignoring my question, types something into the phone, smiles, and walks out of the room. I take that as my cue to leave.

I get in my car, open my phone, and see a message from Mona. She had been texting me! It says, "Figure it out yourself. Oh . . . and namaste."

The next morning, I light some candles on my altar, roll out my yoga mat, close my eyes, and begin to meditate. My thoughts immediately turn to the children, and I replay in my mind the events from two nights before. My body tenses as I think about how disruptive and disrespectful they were. My mind fantasizes about how I can get out of going back. And then I stop. I remind myself to feel into the tension in my body, breathe into it. I do and wiggle a bit to get more comfortable. I try to keep my attention on my breath, watching the inhalations and exhalations and noticing any thoughts that arise. Acknowledge them and let them pass, I remind myself, don't indulge them. But I can't help myself, and my mind gets caught in an endless loop of replaying what happened and imagining what will happen if I go back. What if they're disruptive? Rude? What if I say something stupid? Harmful? I go down a rabbit hole of doubt and recriminations. Meditation doesn't appear to be working. I open my eyes and focus on what's directly in front of me. My altar is filled with candles, pictures, bronze statues of deities, and found objects—stones and feathers representing earth and sky. The flame from the candle is burning hot, the blue and orange fire pulls me into some form of stillness. I shift my eyes to the small bronze statues I brought back with me from India: Kali, Shiva, Krishna, and Ganesh. I should be absorbing the spiritual direction they offer, but all I notice is the dust they're covered in. I reach forward and wipe each one down with my T-shirt. I rearrange them and move more items around. I pick up a picture of my mother, look at her beautiful face, and hold it to my heart. I instinctively send her love and immediately feel our connection from across the country, time and distance not separating our bond. I have no doubt she can feel me, too. I hope she's having a good day and wish her happiness. My body relaxes into that thought.

Is this praying? I wonder.

I recall what Mona said about praying for the kids, but I'm not sure how. I think back to India and the bee. That was the first time I ever really prayed. I remember asking for guidance, clarity, and illumination. My prayer was definitely answered. Quickly and painfully. I hesitate to be so bold again. It occurs to me that when I pray, I'm asking for something—for myself. A change in attitude, an opening of awareness, a shift in perspective. I don't think I've ever prayed *for* someone else.

I step onto my mat—the place I feel the most comfortable—and figure I'll just see what comes to me. If nothing else, I'll feel better.

I stand and begin my sun salutes. Inhale, arms reach; exhale, fold; inhale, look up and lengthen; exhale, jump back; inhale, Upward Dog; exhale, Downward Dog . . .

The movements are familiar and fluid, and I feel my system settle as I stretch and indulge in the sensations, feeling into the tension, my inhales and exhales deep and resonant. I let myself fall into the rhythm of linking movement with breath.

Holding Downward-Facing Dog, it occurs to me that if everything is connected, that would include the vibration from my body and the intentions that drive my thoughts. Perhaps I can direct positive and loving energy from my body to theirs, to the kids? Perhaps I can send thoughts of respect and caring to them and allow my body to be the physical expression of those thoughts? That seems like a good thing to do.

I jump from Downdog to the front of the mat and stand in Mountain Pose. Feeling my roots and my connection with the earth, I place my palms into namaste.

I hesitate at first, not quite sure what to say, not quite sure whom to pray to. Without thinking any more about it, I hear myself speaking. "Calling in the God of my own understanding, be it my Higher Power, the Creative Consciousness, Mother Earth, or the Holy Mother Herself."

Well, that just about covers it, I think. Now, what is it I'm offering?

"May every movement and each breath of this sacred practice be blessed, and may the energy in my body and the love in my heart reach beyond the here and now, and touch the souls of those tender beings, those beautiful young children, wherever they may be in this moment. I dedicate this practice to the healing of their bodies and souls and to the awakening of their magnificent spirit."

What is it that I wish?

"May they be happy, may they be safe, may they continue to grow and expand their own capacity for love. May they heal and be protected. May they remember always who they truly are and be blessed forevermore for their humanity, their beauty, their innocence, and their light."

And while I'm at it, what about me? What's my part in this?

"May I wake up. May I have the strength to continuing walking this path with clarity and integrity and embrace all I experience as opportunities for growth. Please God, transform my resistance into surrender, my judgment into compassion, and my fear into faith. May this faith be the quality of my being that moves me forward on this journey and may I trust that all that is revealed is for the highest good of my soul. May my heart open to these children. May I learn fully from their wisdom. May they reveal to me both the depth of my ignorance and the power of my love. May I experience that love fully within our infinitely shared Spirit and know that we are One, we are whole, and we are blessed with God's ever-present light. Blessed be."

Okay, I think, *that's a pretty good fucking prayer.*

I begin to move again. Inhale, arms reach; exhale, fold; inhale, look up and lengthen; exhale, jump back; inhale, Upward Dog; exhale, Downward Dog . . .

My practice has awakened. Every movement becomes a dedication and an expression of my love. I feel it deep in my body. The way I place my hands onto the floor, the way I arrange my feet, the rhythm of my breath—all become part of an embodied ritual that churns stagnant, caustic energy into something new, powerful, and magickal. Magick with a *k* is different from magic without one. Magic is pulling a rabbit out of a hat or creating illusions that can ultimately be explained. Magick is an ancient hermetic form of spiritual practice that includes ritual and ceremony. My dear friend Damien Echols, who authored the book *High Magick*, describes it as "directing energy using the will." That's exactly what I'm doing and have been doing since the moment I stepped onto my first mat; I just didn't realize it until now. The tension becomes release, the contraction expansion, the judgment understanding, the resentment acceptance. Alchemically, yoga transforms the lead of our fear into the gold of our love. It is magick.

At the end of my practice, I sit tall in meditation, still and quiet. I am present. I rest in the stillness found in the gap between the exhale and the inhale. No beginning, no end. My eyes turn upward as I turn inward.

After a long while, I open my eyes. The candles on my altar still flicker. The deities bear witness. My mother's face still smiles, her eyes holding my own, which are now filled with tears. I get it. No . . . it's more than that. I *feel* it. It wasn't the children's rage or anger that scared me. It was what was underneath. Grief. I was afraid of their sadness, just as I have long been afraid of my own.

Rage masks their deep pain, just as it has cloaked mine. Compassion wells up in my heart. I breathe it into me, into them, and into our shared trauma. Even though our experiences aren't the same, many of the results are—shame, fear, sadness, and most certainly distrust.

I take another deep breath in and sit with the grief—theirs and my own. I now know that moving through grief, being vulnerable in this way, is what leads to freedom, which leads to surrender, and surrender is what opens us to God.

I know who these children are, and I know that I must be in service to them. Lord knows, they will be in service to me, too.

Your pain is your purpose . . . Mona's voice echoes in my head.

I smile and then remember the rest of that thought.

. . . and the true revolution to freedom begins the moment we answer the soul's call for peace.

For the rest of the week, I dedicate my practice to those kids, sending them love, respect, and healing energy, and I ask for clarity, confidence, commitment, surrender, and guidance each time I place my palms in prayer so I may know how best to serve. It becomes clear to me that yoga is so many different things and can be experienced in many ways, but on my mat, in this way, with conscious intention and mindful movement, my practice is a prayer. It aligns me—body, mind, and Spirit—with the whole of the Universe in interdependence . . . and empathy.

Come the following Tuesday, I show up at the shelter again, and find myself back in the common room where the kids are once again sprawled out, watching TV. The session plays out pretty much like it did the week before, but this time I stay grounded and refuse to react, no matter how rude or disruptive they are. *Don't personalize this,* I think. *Meet fear with love. No matter what. Remember who they are to you.* Each week I continue to show up. Each week I roll out my mat and do my best to teach them to breathe and get into their bodies.

After a few months, I sit down with the director, and we discuss my experience at the shelter and the challenges I've been facing with the kids. I tell her my own personal story and ask if it would be okay if I share some of it with them. I tell her I hope that by being honest about my own journey and challenges, the youth and I might connect with each other on a different level. She agrees, provided that the counselors are present in case anything comes up. Driving home, I think about how I will share my story and how, perhaps, if I can offer it up without any shame or judgment, I can *show* them the power of yoga, rather than teach it.

The following week the kids greet me with their customary groans. Instead of insisting they move to their mats, however, I walk over to where they are and sit down. They look so perplexed when I tell them I have something to share with them that they immediately sit up and turn off the TV. I take a deep breath and tell my story. I begin with an abbreviated version of what happened to me as a child, my OCD, my acting out with drugs, alcohol, stealing, and sex. And then I explain how yoga helped me to heal, make healthier choices, manage big feelings and anxiety, and not freak out when the shit was hitting the fan.

The kids listen, some nodding their heads, especially when I bring up my OCD. I already knew some of them had it, having recognized the different forms of patterning they were using to self-regulate. I also saw multiple self-inflicted cut marks on a few arms and legs, where knives or razor blades had been pressed into the skin. When I share how I used to cut my feet until they bled and be obsessed with fours and eights, they're astonished. They can't believe I'm "weird" like that too. One of the youngest ones is particularly surprised by my confession. "You're rich, right? And you're white. Do bad things like this happen to rich, white people, too?" I can tell she genuinely believes that privilege exempts people from pain and suffering. I take that in, suddenly realizing the complexity of that question. I'm not sure what to say. The counselors interject and assure her that abuse doesn't discriminate . . . but neither does healing.

"How about some yoga now?" I ask them. They agree. But this time I invite them to move however they want. They can mimic my movements, do their own thing, or lie on the floor and do nothing. I practice with them side by side, so they can see my body and hear my breathing. I don't instruct. I just remind them to breathe, stretch, and express what they feel in their bodies—in their own way. I encourage them to take ownership of their body in whatever way feels right for them. They do—

reluctantly at first. Then, one of the kids jumps up and turns on some music. Missy Elliott comes blasting through the room—and the kids come alive. They start to sing along, and before I know it, they've pulled me off my mat, and all of us, including the counselors, are dancing, moving our bodies wildly through the space, and singing at the top of our lungs to "Work It."

When the song ends, the teens are in a heap on the floor, all smiling and exhausted. I invite them all to lie down on their mats and close their eyes, if they wish. Then I guide them to relax each body part, starting with their head and moving down the body to their feet. The counselors sit nearby. We share in the sweetness of this moment as the children, one by one, drift off into sleep. They are, for now, completely safe from harm.

As I sit there taking it all in, I know this is where I am meant to serve and that service is my reason for being. Without a doubt, this is yoga in action. This is what it means to take my yoga off the mat and into the world. I also know that this is just the beginning—I have so much to learn. I put my hands in prayer and silently say to the children, "I see you because I AM you. There is no separation. We are One." Then I add, "Show me, God, all that I don't see. Show me the differences, show me my ignorance, so that I may take accountability for how I still create the separation I say I want healed." I sigh. I know I've just opened a portal into a new level of inquiry. I only hope I have the strength to enter and the willingness to embrace all that it will reveal.

I slowly speak the children awake and bring them up into meditation. We sit quietly together, eyes closed and breath soft. *Oh Mona, you are so right. Our pain is our purpose, and a revolution springs from that realization* . . . a revolution of awakened souls, united in heart, aligned with God, in service to each other, the planet, and the Divine. And if all beings could come together and do what needs to be done, in empathy, there would be peace, and we would all, finally, be free.

TEACHINGS FROM THE CHILDREN
SERVICE, PRAYER, AND PURPOSE

By the time I'd been teaching yoga for several years, I felt ready to put my yoga into action, through conscious and compassionate service. I wanted to fix what was broken, heal what was wounded. I just knew the shelter would be a perfect place to share my passion.

Sadly, it wasn't—not at first. Instead, what happened that first week was no different from what had happened at all the rallies and protests I had attended earlier in my life—it was just quieter, more intimate. I once again, inadvertently, set up an "us versus them" polarity. I saw the youth as victims, traumatized and broken, who needed to be "fixed," and I saw myself appearing   seemingly out of nowhere—with a toolbox of "solutions" with which to fix them: do yoga, breathe deeply, meditate daily. To them, I probably came across as just another entitled white woman assuaging her own guilt by volunteering her time in a place where she didn't belong, with people she could never understand.

My first mistake was to think that what worked for me would automatically work for them. I came equipped with sequences and breathing techniques that had changed my life and a whole spiel about the power of yoga, all of which was met with skepticism and plenty of eye rolls. What the hell was wrong with them, anyway? Yoga can help them—I can help them—and if they'd only listen, if they'd only do as I ask, they'd get it. Obviously, *I* didn't get it. I didn't get that yoga is more than a set of class plans, more than my personal experience, that yoga's power is in its ability to change and adapt and meet the needs of the population it's serving. I couldn't meet the needs of these young people as long as I failed to see the differences between me and them. As long as I failed to understand *why* they refused to close their eyes when I asked them to, why even talking about their bodies made them so uncomfortable that they giggled and squirmed. These were children who had endured unfathomable abuse, been stripped of any sense of control, and suffered unimaginable trauma. Why would they, why should they, trust a stranger?

The thing is service requires compassionate action, and compassionate action requires connection. My actions created separation instead. Not because I couldn't relate to the kids, but because I related too much. They *were* me—and that freaked me out. I encountered fifteen raging examples of my disowned and shadow self, and in that moment my yoga—and everything I believed—was put to the test. It didn't do so well. I got completely overwhelmed. And scared. Scared of what? Scared of being out of control. Scared of what I don't understand. Scared of big feelings—theirs and mine. Scared of feeling inadequate. Scared of being dismissed, made fun of. Scared for the wounded little girl in me. Because of my fears, I couldn't truly see them, and I couldn't fully serve them. I would have done well to listen to Carl Jung, who said, "The best political, social, and spiritual work we can do is withdraw the projections of our shadow onto others." If we don't, our shadow will hide the truth of our soul and prevent us from seeing the soul's truth in others.

THE ESSENTIAL TRUTH

Yoga teaches us that the biggest stumbling block to connection is our inability, or unwillingness, to see the truth, to see things as they are—and this is the important part—*without distortion*, without ego interference. This is *satya*. The truth is pure and unchangeable; it's not open to interpretation—emotional or intellectual. In fact, to get to the truth, you must transcend the ego and let the soul speak. You must pay attention! Satya is more than simply saying what is true; it is *living* our truth. Satya is our purest essence, our basic goodness, our highest Self. It is the God within.

I was clearly not "in my truth" that first day at the shelter. I only saw the children through the lens of my own suffering. I saw them as broken because I saw myself as broken. I saw them as something to fear because they were everything that I fear I am. I closed my eyes without ever seeing what was in front of me, I opened my mouth without ever listening, and I delivered my message without once understanding how any of it would be received.

As a result, I came with a yogic prescription that worked for me, blithely assuming it would work for them too. It didn't. But their version of yoga did. As soon as they cranked up the music, I got it. This is yoga; this is the language they understand; this is the medicine that can help heal them. And in heeding their invitation to take a taste of what they were offering, I saw that it had the power to heal me as well.

PAIN IS YOUR PURPOSE

The Dalai Lama once said, "Those you hate [or who scare you] the most are your greatest teachers." And boy, was he right. Those kids at the shelter *were* my teachers, and their teachings humbled me to my core. Mona had said much the same thing: "Our pain is our purpose." And so did Buddhist teacher Thich Nhat Hanh: "Through suffering we learn compassion and understanding." So, who better than me to work alongside young children who had experienced trauma because of sexual exploitation and abuse? Who

better than those teenagers to force me to welcome all parts of myself and accept those same parts in them? To cultivate empathy and compassion for their suffering and my own? My pain, my purpose. Full fucking circle.

If you have experienced trauma, when you've done your own healing work and the time is right, ask yourself the same questions. Who better than you to stand in the presence of another soul with empathy, based on your own journey? Who better than you to know what is possible? Who better than you to know the ways in which the other person wants to run, hide, sabotage, and resist? Who better than you to know what's on the other side of that resistance? This wisdom doesn't come from books; it is earned through the hardship of being and the deep release that comes from surrender. This empathy, grounded in a shared understanding, is what can heal a soul through recognition—yours and theirs.

And don't think for a moment that you have to have experienced trauma in your life in order to be of service to others. You don't. If you are someone who is moving through life without a lot of hardship—challenges, yes, just not the unmanageable kind—you'll still need to face your fears, biases, and privileges, anything that stands in your way of serving others. Because here's the thing. You cannot connect with someone whose behaviors you find abhorrent in yourself or whose situation you fail or refuse to understand. Do the inner work and then get off your ass and serve. To not do so is to ignore the obvious suffering around you. That doesn't necessarily make you a bad person, but it does make you complicit in the continued plight and oppression of others. Just sayin'.

The challenges we've gone through can help us be more compassionate and connected or, if we're not careful, it can close our minds and keep us separate. Then what do we do? Once again, Thich Nhat Hanh nails it so poetically. We must "learn the art of taking good care of our suffering so we can learn the art of transforming it." What does that mean? It means treating our wounds with tenderness and understanding and seeing the whole of our being—*as it is*. I learned how to see, feel, and discharge my big emotions—from Mona and trauma work as well as asana, meditation, and prayer. And then—here's the important part—the journey must continue outward. Our inner work must inform our outer work, our dharma. Only then can we meet those we wish to serve with our full attention, employing all of our senses so we may hear, see, and feel into *their* experience and meet them where they are. It's always easier to be compassionate and forgiving toward someone or something we know intimately.

LIVING YOUR DHARMA

Dharma is living life on purpose, whether that purpose is born from pain or arises out of a special talent you wish to share with others. Dharma comes into play, as Deepak Chopra says, when "we blend this unique talent in service to others," and we experience "the ecstasy and exultation of our own spirit, which is the ultimate goal of all goals."

Dharma is the soul's work, the truest expression of who you are. It emerges from the depth of your wisdom body, your heart-mind; it is the universe guiding you to your purpose and your willingness to surrender to its call. To see the soul in another and to shine your light in the world for the benefit of all beings—that is what you're here in this body to do. Remember that the soul wants experience because it's through experience, through connection, that consciousness can evolve.

The good news is you don't have to have it all together to step into that purpose. As Krishna tells Arjuna in the Bhagavad Gita, "It is better to live your own dharma imperfectly, than to live an imitation of somebody else's life with perfection." You may never transcend your ego or scrub your shadow self clean. Serve anyway. Your work is to show up *as you are*—without denying, burying, or justifying your shadow emotions—and then commit to serving consciously and in love, as best you can.

Your shadow can lead you to your purpose, if you're willing to learn from it and see its usefulness. I think author and activist Parker Palmer said it best when he addressed the 2015 graduating class at Naropa University: "Take everything that is bright and beautiful in you and introduce it to the shadow side of yourself. Let your altruism meet your egoism, let your generosity meet your greed, let your joy meet your grief . . . but when you are able to say 'I am all of the above, my shadow as well as my light,' the shadow's

power is put in service to the good." And you have found your dharma.

When you accept your dharma, you commit to a life of truth—of satya—and vow to participate in the liberation of all souls. You come to understand, as the Buddha taught, that you can never be free until all souls are free. And what is that freedom? Samadhi. Samadhi means "seeing equally"; experiencing life as it is, in the present moment, without wanting things to be different, without clinging to the past or anticipating the future. It is putting aside your ego, your identities, and resting in a state of *being* instead of *doing*. In his classic *Light on Life*, B.K.S. Iyengar said we get a glimpse of samadhi in Savasana, which he says is the most difficult yoga posture of all because it invites us to simply *be* without being the someone who *is*, to shed all our "prejudices, preconceptions, ideas, memories, and projects for the future" and reside in our true nature. It is Billy's invitation to ignore the story and see the soul in all beings and remember to love. See the soul, and you will meet yourself. Meet yourself, and you will know God. Know God, and you will experience love. Be that love, and you will know liberation.

So serve where you are called. Serve in a way that is sustainable. Be open to what presents itself. Service may look completely different from how you thought it would look. Serve anyway. Just give of yourself in benefit to the happiness, good will, safety, abundance, and ease of others . . . and watch your own heart open in unimaginable ways.

PRAYER AS SERVICE

It's hard to serve others when the noise of your own shadow drowns out the cries of someone else's suffering. And that's how it was for me and the children I was trying to serve. We can't understand what we fail to see, feel, or hear. Serving others requires deep listening, the ability to feel energy and connect to its vibrations in a way that will benefit others, not harm them. I was too reactive to listen, too vulnerable to see and feel. When Mona told me to pray for those kids, I had no idea what she meant or how to do that. But I did know how to work with energy.

Yoga teaches that everything we think, feel, and experience—and everything we have ever thought, felt, and experienced—is energy and is governed by the pranamaya kosha (the energy body). Remember, energy is vibration that carries within it information. If my thoughts are negative, the energy I create and project outward will be negative too. If my thoughts are positive, the energy I project will be positive, creating an aura of loving-kindness. Just like diet and environment, the energy circulating through me—from my thoughts, perceptions, and ideas—affects the health of my body and the clarity of my mind. It is also possible to direct this energy, in a positive *or* negative way, to others—through touch, words, and even thoughts. Since we are all connected and bound by energy, it makes sense that we would all be impacted by what flows between us as well.

I came to understand that prayer is energy, a way to connect with the highest resonance, or vibration, within us. Praying can be a way to focus that energy on a question or problem we need more clarity or insight around. We pray to align ourselves with God, to come into harmony with a frequency that is higher than the low-density vibration of our physical body. We are already capable of connecting to these higher frequencies, but our ego and the challenges of living in the physical world dim the light and restrict our ability to access it.

Prayers can also be a way to acknowledge what it is you want and desire, and to ask for wisdom, clarity, and acceptance as you open yourself to receive, knowing that however the prayer is answered—and it may be completely different from what you hoped for—will ultimately be the guidance you need for your growth.

Praying for someone else means taking in energetic abundance—the goodwill and love within your own energetic body—and offering it out to someone or something that needs it. Praying that they receive all that they need, which may include forgiveness, healing, acceptance, and surrender. Again, you can't control anyone's destiny, but you can align your heart with theirs and hold them in the sacred space of your being. A side effect of offering such thoughts is the well-being that it brings, the sense of being connected. And when you feel more connected, it changes your relationship to the day, to the people you encounter, and even to the work you do. You become a living prayer, seeing the sacred in all things and all things in the sacred.

Aligning heart-to-heart awakens our intuitive mind so we can remember how to empathize. Empathy, of course, is different from sympathy. Sympathy (which means "feeling in common") is concern from the sidelines, with no internal connection, and often implies judgment (*I feel bad for you; you poor thing, it must suck*). It's understanding from an intellectual point of view. *I've been there; I know what you're going through.* Empathy (which means "feeling into") is a visceral reaction to something someone else is going through; it's experiencing it as the other person—*I feel your pain; I am right there with you.* Compassion (to feel with, to suffer with) is empathy laced with the desire to alleviate the other person's suffering.

BODY-BASED PRAYER

I couldn't empathize with the young people at the shelter as long as I erected barriers between us. In order to connect, Mona said I needed to pray, but I didn't know how—not until I allowed my body to teach me. I began to move because that's what I know, that's what I do, that's how I listen. Each day I would put my palms together and dedicate each movement, every breath to those young people. I could see them, feel them; I could hold both their suffering and healing in my heart and allow the energy from the prayer to move through me and into them. I asked for guidance, strength, and patience for myself. I asked for protection, ease, and well-being for them. My practice became a meditation in action, an offering beyond the body, and a ritual meant to align my heart with theirs in love. The barriers became more porous until they disappeared completely. I called my practice "body prayer," and it united me with them and in Spirit as undifferentiated and whole.

When we offer our practice as prayer, yoga becomes its own act of service, an expression of our activism that requires no additional expenditure, monetary or otherwise—just focus, generosity of heart, unwavering love, and abiding devotion.

Once I began to pray, my practice became more of an energetic one, capable of taking me into higher states of transformative awareness. I felt like a priestess, collecting energy, charging it with positive intentions, and then directing it outward—my limbs likes wands—onto my intended

recipients. This magick helped me see yoga's influence on the whole and to understand that the way in which we participate in or hold space for change matters. Prayer matters. Energy matters. Connection matters. Love matters. And it is one more way we can serve this world into healing.

ANSWERING THE CALL

When Mona said, "Your pain is your purpose," she added this: "and the true revolution to freedom begins the moment we answer the soul's call for peace." What does that even mean? We are all being asked to show up, find our voice, take action, honor life, participate in growth, and BE the motherfucking change! That's what she was talking about. *This* is the revolution of the soul! Don't turn away from your humanity; turn toward it. Don't bypass your shadow emotions—learn from them, uncover the wisdom within them. By looking at yourself with honesty and clarity, you can tear down the walls that separate you from those you wish to serve. For it is collective growth, moving from fear into love, that will guide our nation, our planet, toward peace. It just will. Love regenerates itself. It sees itself in ALL. It cannot separate or cause pain and suffering. When we let our purpose move us into action, with the compassion, acceptance, and care that brought us to our own healing, we can show others, through the words, deeds, and choices we make, what waking up can look like and how it can benefit all beings. This is the revolution that inspires change—from the inside out. It is sustainable. It is meaningful. It is sacred. It is whole, and it is ours to behold, embody, and activate. We can't wait for anyone to answer the call for us. *We* are the leaders. "We," as the poet June Jordan said, "are the ones we have been waiting for."

For years, I prayed to wake up. Service was, and continues to be, the answer to that prayer and my greatest teacher. It exposes the deep ignorance, bias, prejudice, and fear embodied within me that keep me separate from, and complicit in, the suffering and inequality of others. My experience at the shelter helped me see that my dharma was to step into conscious leadership and contribute to social change as an expression of yoga in action. Turns out I had much to learn about what that meant. Recognizing the ways in which those children and I were the same helped me see them, but understanding the ways in which we were different ultimately helped me serve them.

Yoga suggests that if you want to change the world, start with yourself. I thought I got that. But, as you'll see, my journey was, and is, far from over. As Nikki Myers put it, "This shit's about to get real, for real."

10

SHOWING UP IN LOVE

VOLUNTEERING AT THE SHELTER initiated me into the next level of my spiritual practice. It opened my eyes to the power of yoga beyond what I had experienced while moving, breathing, and chanting all those years on my mat. It was no longer just about me—*my* health, *my* healing, *my* happiness. I knew beyond a shadow of a doubt that yoga can change lives and open hearts. And it does that by adapting its gifts to the needs of the population it is serving. Once I got that—in truth, once the young people at the shelter *taught* me that—I couldn't wait to share this sacred practice with the world. I was ready to serve humanity, and I jumped into that calling with my whole heart and soul.

By the early 2000s, yoga had hit the big time, veering away from its spiritual roots and landing squarely in the fitness world. All over the West, people were rolling out their mats and stepping into Downward Dog on the daily, often with a soy latte positioned within reach and always with perfectly fitting color-coordinated leggings. I didn't care if the only reason someone wanted to do yoga was to tone their abs or tighten their butt. My experience taught me that in time and with commitment, yoga would guide each soul into a personal awakening beyond the body. I was happy to see so many people, who might normally shy away from a practice steeped in spirit, step onto their mats.

As a white, fit, young woman with a riot of curly hair that made me instantly recognizable, I was well positioned to benefit from all this mainstreaming. And benefit I did—with corporate sponsorships and video deals, magazine covers and feature stories. Through hard work, luck, and the opportunities that come from being marketable, I became what people called a "rock star" yogi. I was traveling, getting lots of attention, and making a living at what I loved best, and that felt good.

But my yogic fame felt good for a deeper reason: it allowed me to fulfill my dharma on a broader scale. I had come to understand that yoga has never been about the stretch; it's always been about the reach. And if I could use my reach to bring yoga's healing powers to people everywhere and my influence to raise awareness and funds for social causes that alleviate suffering and separation, then I was all in.

I did all sorts of volunteering, working with sex-trafficked youth in the US, the Women's Action Coalition, and other organizations. I became the national yoga ambassador for YouthAIDS, which provided services for children worldwide effected and affected by HIV/AIDS. To raise money for their efforts, I created T-shirts that said "Off the Mat, Into the World" and sold them for twenty bucks. I raised a hundred thousand dollars in just a few months. Damn. That was easy. People in my community wanted to help. I was clearly onto something.

I began teaching workshops on spiritual activism around the country as a way of combining my love of yoga and my desire to serve, which I saw as essential steps on the path toward liberation. My students were eager to explore the topic, and the workshops were a success. Between raising funds so effortlessly and seeing the enthusiasm of my students, I began to imagine a movement of global yogis committing to their dharma, creating change, raising money, and working together in service to each other, the planet, and God.

Problem was I didn't know how to make that happen alone. I didn't have the resources, skills, or experience to organize any kind of a movement, let alone one that could harness the mainstream yoga community. I needed to partner with people I knew who shared a similar vision and explore with them the ways in which we could collaborate.

So, in 2007, my dear friends Hala Khouri and Suzanne Sterling and I started Off the Mat, Into the World (OTM). OTM is a leadership training program designed to help people bridge the gap between yoga's transformational power and the imperative of social justice and action. We wanted to train people from all over the country, helping them step into purpose and leadership in their own local community. We also started the Global Seva Challenge, where students were invited to raise twenty thousand dollars to support various grassroot organizations around the world that were doing extraordinary work with folks on the margins. If the students succeeded, they would get to visit and work with the organizations and see firsthand how the money was being spent. OTM split the money the students collected among all the organizations and then used my media connections to create awareness and draw attention to the organizations' work.

With all this in mind, I traveled first to South Africa, where I visited several organizations dedicated to eradicating HIV/AIDS and then on to Uganda. Focusing on HIV/AIDS, in my mind, was a meaningful way to honor Billy and the impact he'd had on my life. I was particularly interested in visiting an orphanage in Uganda, which housed and provided care for children affected by HIV/AIDS. The disease was (and still is) very prevalent throughout that part of the country; many children were either living with HIV/AIDS themselves, having been born with the disease, or they had become heads of their own households, after their parents or grandparents (or, more often than not, both) died from it. The orphanage was also a permaculture farm, where the children learned to work the land and obtain the skills that would hopefully provide income for their future.

What I was about to discover was that the best intentions can create unintended consequences. That overseas "service" trips like these can often be problematic and, even worse, create more division. Here's what happened.

▼

I arrive at the farm and am greeted warmly by dozens of laughing and playful children. Two grab hold of my hands and lead me through the front gates to a large, pristine farm, with dung-colored buildings dotted along the property. They're excited to show me the land and their work. They describe what permaculture is, how every resource is used and shared, and how nothing gets wasted. One small boy takes great delight in explaining to me how they even use chicken poop to paint the white fence—the very one I am leaning against!

We gather for dinner in the main house, a large wooden structure that doubled as a school room during the day. The young people have prepared a vegan meal from the vegetables grown on their land. It seems like every person on the farm is here, their voices loud and animated as some of the children speak to each other, and others practice their English with me.

After the food is served, the director of the farm, Tibyangye Ntende, walks into the room and takes his place at the table. He's from the community, and through the practice of permaculture farming and seed sharing, has helped elevate six neighboring villages, including his own, from poverty. He smiles and says a warm "Hello!" to the folks gathered and then introduces himself to me, clasping my hand with both of his. He looks around and comments on how beautiful the food looks—almost as beautiful as everyone in the room, he adds—and smiles at the children as they giggle and blush. He then asks us all to join hands. The room grows silent as everyone reaches for a hand to hold. He begins to pray, offering heartfelt words of gratitude for our food, for the community, for each other, and for the endless love of God.

He ends his prayer with "Asante Mungu. Upendo njia zote, kila mara"—Thank you God. May we love all ways, always—which the children repeat back enthusiastically. Then we begin to eat. After a bit of light conversation, Tibyangye looks around the room, taking in the thirty or so of us seated there, winks at me, and with a gentle smile, says, "Children, I have a question for you." The kids stop what they are doing and look expectantly at Tibyangye, who continues, "I'm curious, what did you do today that made you feel happy, excited, or proud?"

Speaking freely and openly, everyone shares little moments that brought them joy, regaling in their accomplishments. The kids listen intently to one another, smiling, clapping, and offering encouragements and congratulations along the way, taking great pleasure in each other's happiness.

Tibyangye is also smiling, giving his full attention to each one. "Wonderful, wonderful!" he keeps saying, and I can tell he genuinely means it. After a while, he speaks again. "Children, I'm curious, what did you do today that you were not proud of or that made you feel angry or ashamed or sad?" No one says a word.

I'm a bit taken aback by the directness of this question and wonder if it is a setup. Did some kid do something wrong? Is this his way of finding the guilty party? I look around the room; almost everyone is staring at their plate.

Then, slowly, the children take turns acknowledging the challenges they faced that day. One child admits that he was mean to another child and made fun of him in front of his friends. He feels guilty and ashamed. The child he had been mean to shares how embarrassed, angry, and hurt he had felt. Then another child, newer to the community, confesses she stole food that morning because she was afraid there might not be any for her in the evening. As she begins to cry, another child, guided by a subtle nod from the director, puts a little more food on the young girl's plate. Everyone listens thoughtfully and encourages each other, especially those who seem particularly vulnerable or reluctant to share.

It is emotional, open, and honest. I am deeply moved.

Tibyangye continues to smile and make eye contact with each child, with no judgment or admonishment in his eyes. Any conflict seems to get resolved among the kids themselves. Forgiveness asked, forgiveness received. He nods his head. "Wonderful, wonderful. Thank you."

Finally, he says, "Children, I have one more question. What will you commit to for tomorrow?"

With that, each child sits up straight and one by one, declares loudly and strongly . . . "Love!"

The word bounces off the wooden walls, floors, and ceiling and becomes a wild and joyous chant. They make it clear to everyone who can hear them. They have committed to love.

I laugh and clap along with the children, then look over at Tibyangye. He holds my gaze for a moment, and then turns his attention back to the children.

After dinner, Tibyangye invites me to walk with him around his farm. As we look at the different gardens and projects, he explains what permaculture is. "In permaculture, everything is used and shared," he says. "Nothing is wasted, and everything supports the other. Its success is dependent on relationships, harmonious relationships, not only with nature, but also with people. If those who tend the animals, dig the ditches, or sow the seeds are out of balance with themselves, each other, spirit, or nature, then it's not permaculture. It might be organic gardening, which has value, but it wouldn't be fully holistic, and therefore, it is not sustainable."

He bends down and picks up a small seed. "The quality of this seed is important, but not more so than the quality of the soil the seed is laid in, which is important, but not more so than the amount of water used to water the seed, which is important . . ." He stops for a moment and looks straight into my eyes, then continues, "but not more so than the quality of the soul of the person digging the hole, planting the seed, watering the crop."

He then says, "Seane, these children have experienced unimaginable trauma. They've lost their families, they are ill, and they have great responsibilities and burdens that beings so young should never know. They deal with the stigma of a disease they had nothing to do with contracting except for simply being born. These children have experienced isolation, abandonment, judgment, and a level of fear that you and I can't really understand."

We walk without speaking for a few moments, absorbed in the sounds of the countryside all around us. He squats down and begins pulling dirt from the red earth, making a hole, then continues. "When the children come here, they are often shy and feel ashamed of their circumstances. They don't trust us; they certainly don't trust me. Why should they? What evidence do they have for kindness and acceptance? We need them to get comfortable with who they are and all that they feel because if they don't, odds are, they will either continue to withdraw from society or act out in other ways. We understand that before they can be in relationship with us, or each other, or this planet, they need to be in harmonious relationship with themselves."

When the hole is deep enough, he buries the seed and pulls the earth over it, patting it down firmly.

"By helping them to become comfortable identifying and sharing their feelings, they can see that others feel the same or similar ways. That their feelings, either good or bad, are just that. Feelings. Feelings change. Everything changes. Through this shared communication, they begin to see that who they are and the way they show up impacts the growth, health, and happiness of others and nature. This is permaculture."

He stands up, and we walk over to the well; he pulls up a bucket filled with water. He walks back to the mound of earth that now covers the seed and carefully pours water over it.

"This is why I encourage the children to explore their feelings, communicate their truths, take accountability for their experience, and celebrate their participation in the world," he says. "They need to learn to love themselves, all parts of themselves, the good stuff and the not so good; only then can they develop the empathy and compassion needed to love the world and each other."

He places the bucket back into the well, wipes his hands on his pants and, turning to face me directly, says, "Accountability is the key to sustainability, and compassion the doorway to peace. That is what we teach the children here. That is what we practice ourselves."

As we head back toward the main house, I try to digest everything he's been telling me. It's not so different from what I've been taught. I smile. Mona would be so pleased with herself. This is what she has been teaching all along. But to connect it to the earth in such a holistic way? Amazing. Tibyangye gently interrupts my reverie. "I'm curious, Seane, what is your commitment in being here?"

I stop and look at him incredulously. Shaking my head, I say, "To help you and the kids, of course. What you're doing is amazing. This should be taught in all schools, to children all around the world. This is what yoga is all about and everything I believe! Why am I here? I want to serve. I want to help. I want to create change. I have money and influence and a large community who will support me in whatever vision I have. You tell me a project you want created and, believe me, I will make that happen!"

"Thank you, Seane. I feel your passion and enthusiasm, I really do. And I know you want to help, but as much as I appreciate your support, I must decline."

I stare at him in confusion. He just rejected my help?

"You see," he says, "there is only ever one answer to that question. And that answer is 'love.'"

Tibyangye puts his arm across my shoulder and begins walking me back to the parking lot where my car is waiting.

"Go home, Seane. Think about what I said. Come back here when love is your only commitment to being of service. Anything less than that, and you'll just be in our way."

He stops on the pathway to face me, the moon behind him outlining his body. "Stay now," he said, "and we'll teach you how to dig a ditch."

Then, pointing toward my heart, he continues, "Come back committed to love, and we'll show you how to fill that hole."

TEACHINGS FROM UGANDA
UNITY, COMMITMENT, AND SUSTAINABILITY

My trip to the farm gave me a swift, divine ass-kicking and woke me up to what true sustainable service means. Hint: it's not all about me. When Tibyangye asked me why I was there, I wanted to say it was because I felt connected to the farm and to their work; I wanted to say I came to be of service. But really, I just wanted to make everything better; the children had broken my heart, and I couldn't bear to witness their suffering. I wanted to fix what I perceived needed to be mended, including my own heart. In truth, I was just another white, entitled benefactor swooping in to save the day, when the day didn't need to be saved in the first place. I wanted Tibyangye to see me as part of the solution—no, I wanted to *be* the solution. I more than implied that *I* could make things happen for them. *I* had influence. *I* had money. *I* had power. Just ask *me*, and I'll make it happen. No "we" ever crossed my lips—or my mind. It never occurred to me to ask if he'd like my help. Why wouldn't he? Who doesn't

want money and access to resources? Turns out, he didn't—not the way I offered it. Taking my money would be out of alignment with the organization's mission and its efforts, and that was something he was not willing to do.

In my eagerness, my ego jumped in ahead of my heart, and my brain quickly differentiated itself from those I hoped to serve. I was, once again, the "fixer," who had the solution to *their* problems, just like I had been at the shelter back home. Rushing in to fix things without connecting first, it turns out, is the number one shadow of the privileged. It creates a hierarchy, a power dynamic designed to perpetuate oppression, born from a model of charity, rather than true service. As long as I positioned myself as separate from them, any relationship I offered would be disordered and would disrupt the holistic system they had created.

Tibyangye got that right away, of course. But he wanted *me* to see that offering to help and being of service were two different things. Help is born from inequality; it is a one-sided offering that puts the helper in a position of authority and those who've been helped forever in the helper's debt. Had I truly come to serve, I would have come in love, with mutual respect, understanding, and a willingness to learn and be useful. The fact that I wanted to give money was not the issue. The fact that I saw my money as the solution to their problems was.

The unequal power dynamics I had inadvertently created as a white woman of privilege—from the United States, no less—perpetuated a sense of "otherness" that was divisive and unsustainable. Those dynamics gave me the freedom to live my life however I chose, oblivious to the ways in which my choices caused harm to others. I clearly wasn't part of the solution; in fact, I was part of the problem. And the problem is that these power differentials continue to fracture the soul of this planet, and her people, because they lead to stealing from the majority for the ease of the few. After Tibyangye's kind but firm take-down, I retreated to reflect on how—after all the inner work I had done and the places I had served—I had made such

a critical misstep. What I was doing served my own comfort, but did little to benefit those I came to serve. What I offered, in the way that I did, clearly was not permaculture—and it certainly wasn't yoga.

A MORE BALANCED DYNAMIC

In some ways, permaculture is the perfect outward manifestation of yoga. Permaculture, as Tibyangye taught me, depends on us creating a harmonious relationship with nature. If we are to heal one another, we must commit to healing the earth; if we are to heal the earth, we must begin with ourselves. The farm's mission was to replace a disordered system, one that had contributed to the ancestral and birth traumas these young children faced, with an ordered system, one in which the children had a chance to heal, grow, and support one another—and, even more important, a system in which the children participated in their own healing and growth.

In permaculture, as well as in yoga and other Eastern traditions, everything is connected, and nothing exists in isolation. When you hold a flower in your hand and look at it, you can see the distinct parts of that flower—the petals, the stem, the leaves, the stamen, and so on—none of which is, by itself, the flower. A flower, obviously, is the sum total of all its pieces. And, it's much more than that. Take a moment, really peer inside the flower, and you will see: the seed it came from, the soil it grew out of, and the water and the sunshine that nourished it. Look even closer, and you will see the person who planted the seed, tilled the soil, and lovingly cared for it. Stay awhile and underneath all that, you'll see that person's parents and grandparents—and all the decisions and experiences in their lives that led them to their purpose. As Tibyangye patiently explained, no single element in nature is more important than any other; every one of them is vital to the flower's existence.

In order to enter into a harmonious relationship with the natural world in a way that creates, nourishes, and sustains, we humans must get our act together. We cannot give back to Mother Earth with the loving attention she deserves and requires if we are emotionally fractured. We can plant stuff, garden organically even, as Tibyangye said. But until we are willing to take ownership of our shadow as well as our light—which, for many of us, includes our internalized privilege and sense of entitlement—we will only succeed in creating more harm. And, sadly, we will be unable to bear witness to the mystery of the natural world and drink from the elixir Nature provides. The kindness and compassion Tibyangye modeled for the children helped them discover their own gifts, rejoice in the gifts of others, and, as a collective, share those gifts with Mother Earth—practical skills, present-moment attention, tender loving care—to create abundance for *all*. In return, Nature gifted them with food for their bodies and beauty and wonderment for their souls.

Tibyangye and his organization did not stumble upon permaculture by accident. Permaculture afforded them a way to create order out of chaos, to literally move from a disordered system that contributed to great suffering and destruction to an ordered one that provided everyone with an equal opportunity to be heard, to be healthy, and to be safe. I began to understand, in retrospect, that this could be applied everywhere. It's so easy to despair that an entire culture, government, and education system—in other words, the systems that determine our reality—are fixed. That there's no way to mend what has been broken for hundreds of years. Tibyangye showed us that this is not true. Systems are made up of people. Change the people—and the way they live and relate to one another—and we can change the system.

YOGA IN ACTION

My own yoga practice epitomizes the evolution from organic gardening to permaculture. Over the years, it has gone from just scratching the surface (tending the garden) to excavating what lay beneath. When I first started yoga, it was all about the physical body—how it felt, its areas of tension, resistance, and openness. I dug a little deeper and discovered if I just breathed a certain way, I could change how my body moved and how it felt. Deeper still, when I held poses longer, I noticed feelings and thoughts that surfaced seemingly out of nowhere. When I fully committed to self-reflection and self-discovery, I saw within me everything and everyone that came before—their pain and sorrows, joys and loves, even their biases and prejudices. It was then I realized that to become whole, to *be love*, I needed to be in relationship with all of that, all of me. It was then I vowed to do the inner work required to awaken to my highest Self. No matter how humbling.

Yoga gives us the capacity to approach the natural world and one another with reverence and a willingness to listen, to show up more from our wisdom mind and less from our logical, "let me tell you what you need" brain. In both permaculture and yoga, living in harmony with all includes ourselves and other people, of course, as well as our animal friends, trees, plants, soil, water, and air. This relationship is divinely bound and sacred.

COME BACK WITH LOVE

When Tibyangye asked me what my commitment was, he wasn't asking how long they could count on my money or how much influence I had. He was asking whether I could commit to love, to being a part of a system that brings harmony, not division, into the world, one that heals the planet as well as the body and the soul of every human being. This kind of love was deeper than the feel-goods I got being around the children, hearing their laughter, seeing how they cared for one another and for themselves. This kind of love comes from the depth of our soul—not from our ego—and it knows no bounds. It's the kind of love that Ancient Greeks, along with Christian theologians including Rev. Dr. Martin Luther King Jr. called *agape*, meaning the highest form of love: selfless, unconditional, "the love of God operating in the human heart."

The yogic path to agape is through selfless service (often called *seva* or karma yoga), which B.K.S. Iyengar said, "is [our] righteous duty [to] uphold, sustain, and support our humanity." But it can only be so if it is infused with *sadhana*, or daily spiritual practice. Sadhana ensures you approach everything you do through a spiritual lens, from the truth of your soul; it is what makes your seva truly selfless.

Permaculture *is* sadhana. It's prayer in action. It's connecting to everything with our full attention and from the heart. From the way we prepare the soil and plant the seed to how we honor and celebrate all the elements that help it grow; from the way we harvest and use what we've planted to the way we do our own physical, emotional, and spiritual work. But I wasn't doing any of that. My dharma was definitely "grounded in purpose," *my* purpose, but not in prayer and not in a willingness to look at my shadow self. It served my unconscious need to be the savior, but that's about it. I held onto the fruits of my actions instead of surrendering them to the greater good and allowing God to speak and act through me. In other words, I had neglected to do my own sadhana in preparation for serving others.

A PERSONAL SADHANA

A daily sadhana is the personal practice you do each day to ground, connect, and reaffirm your commitment to your highest Self and to love. It's your personal prayer. Sadhana is best done early in the morning, when the world is quiet and you have yet to step into your day. But if the start of your day doesn't include early morning, you can begin your sadhana at any time.

Sadhana brings mindfulness into everything you do and say—the way you brush your teeth and brew your coffee or tea; the way you move into and out of your asana postures, placing your attention in that special way vinyasa invites us to do; the way you prepare your food, the foods you choose, and how you eat; the way you interact with the people you meet, the conversations you have, the listening you're able to commit to, and the accountability you're willing to take.

A very basic sadhana may be one that includes some gentle stretches, several minutes of pranayama, a little longer meditation, and a walk in nature, all of which support your nervous system, clear your mind, and allow you to move through your day a bit more consciously. A deeper commitment may include prayer in which you ask the question *What do I need to do to get to the truth, to align myself with the God within?*, and a body-based meditation in which you listen into the silence and receive the answers. After a particularly focused practice or sit, you may feel a sense of calm abiding within you, like I did that day so many years ago in front of the Greenwich Avenue clock. Serving from that place of unity can help keep the ego in check or, as Parker Palmer says, put its power "in service to the good."

Sadhana is permaculture for your soul, and it puts your prayers into action. It was what helped me summon my inner wisdom at the shelter in LA when I needed it most and awakened my empathy and compassion. You may want to pray that you can bring all the principles of yoga into your daily life: that you are able to approach others in ways that do no harm (ahimsa); that you can show up in truth (satya), a truth not obscured by your own desires or hampered by your ego; that you don't take what doesn't belong to you or appropriate what you can't understand (asteya)—not only tangible objects but, more important, other people's stories and other people's experiences.

PUTTING SADHANA INTO PRACTICE

Unfortunately, my time at the farm was not my finest dharma hour. I bypassed the sadhana part (the *being*) and plunged headfirst into action (the *doing*) without even asking what needed to be done. I forgot another golden rule of both yoga and permaculture: observe first. In the immortal words of Donna Summer, we must stop, look, and listen—before we act. I knew all this, of course, but my desire to rush in and be the one who saved the day overrode my ability to stop, look, *or* listen. I had observed what was happening *around* me, but I hadn't observed what was happening *within* me. I wasn't coming from a place of wholeness or balance when I swooped in to serve "others." I had forgotten that there is no "other" to serve—no separation between me and those children or anyone else; no separation between me and the water, trees, plants, soil, and air; no separation between me and our animal friends, the ones easy to love and the creepy-crawly ones that may sometimes give us pause. No separation, literally, not just figuratively. This is not just an intellectual nod to a theoretical truth. It *is* truth.

And yet . . .

Our world thrives on dualities, our systems depend upon it, and participating in separation has become so normalized that it feels as natural as breathing. Although I always wanted to believe that we are all One, united in a shared humanity, my experiences in Uganda and elsewhere made me question those beliefs. I certainly didn't need to travel halfway across the world to see that so much was dictated by race, class, upbringing, education, and culture. How could unity ever be possible with things so polarized? I was going to have to unpack all that in my own heart and mind if I was going to participate in creating a just and balanced society for all. But, first, I needed to witness and right the imbalance within me.

How could creating balance within myself help end disparity and division outside myself? Remember, as Tibyangye and his organization proved, we change the system by changing the people who keep it alive—and that change begins with ourselves. Why? First of all, so that we can see where our disharmony contributes to the pain and suffering of others. Secondly, as yoga and permaculture suggest, there is no separation between our inner world and the outer world. We contain within us the same fundamental forces that are found in nature—stability (*tamas*), energy (*rajas*), and harmony or basic goodness (*sattva*)—the *gunas* as they are called in Sanskrit. These three intertwine, in various ways, to create everything (visible and invisible) in the universe and within ourselves as well. All of this weaving together happens without us being conscious of it, but we can learn to pay attention to their individual characteristics so we can figure out how they work and how we can work *with* them.

THE GUNAS IN NATURE AND WITHIN

A sattvic world is one of abundance, beauty, order, and balance. To achieve sattva, things need to get moving, and rajas is the guna that makes that happen. Rajas governs the beginning of the life cycle—during birth and growth. It's what causes a seed to grow into a plant and the plant to flower. Tamas predominates the end of the life cycle; it's the destructive force that causes the plant to break apart, die back, and return to the soil. Sattva is the time in between, when the flower is in full bloom and beauty is all around us. Nothing can live without energy (rajas). There can be no harvest, no beauty without sattva, and there can be no rebirth without tamas. All of nature depends on a healthy relationship between creation and destruction—rajas and tamas—to support the health and vitality of the planet and all who abide there (sattva).

Just like in nature, our physical and mental health depend on the proper interplay among the gunas. When all three gunas are in balance, everything arises (rajas), abides (sattva), and dissolves (tamas)—whether we're talking about the life cycle of a plant, an idea, a pose, or a stage of life. Rajas moves the energy and creates; sattva preserves and abides; tamas disperses and destroys. Rajas is the in-breath; tamas, the out-breath; and sattva, the gap in between—the silence where liberation can happen, where magick resides, and where everything is whole.

Rajas (Active or Distracted)

Rajas provides the passion and desire to get things done and the effort and enthusiasm required to make it all happen. Unfortunately, it can also make you flighty, impatient, and annoying and can create harmful division when left unchecked. Without the steadiness of tamas or the self-awareness of sattva, rajas can cause you to act without thinking, to rush into situations without checking to see how your actions align with those you wish to serve. You may become impatient when others don't see things your way or sign on for stuff when you're already maxed out. Rajas fuels the desire to serve but only to the extent that such service makes you look and feel good; rajas is all about ego gratification. Rajastic types need validation and look for happiness outside themselves. If tamas is self-beat, rajas is self-righteousness. It's acting without listening, serving without connecting. Rajas is privilege run amok—barging in without wondering, asking, or even caring if you're needed; being attached to your own power; and not giving a damn how the system affects others. In my case, excitement and my desire to help bulldozed their way front and center, and I never even saw how I wasn't listening or connecting. If my experience is any indication, rajas at the very least can make us into impatient and presumptuous assholes.

Tamas (Stable or Apathetic)

Tamas brings a sense of inner stability and groundedness, which can stop you from jumping into action prematurely or overextending yourself. When it dominates, however, that stability can turn to apathy, obstruction, and self-beat—*Who am I, thinking I can make a difference? What do I have to offer?*—and keep you from getting off the couch and doing something. It can also cause you to hold fast to your own limiting beliefs. This tamasic lethargy dulls the mind, which can prevent you from understanding what is happening or seeing how your actions, unearned advantages, biases, and deep-seated traumas contribute to the suffering of others—and of yourself.

Tamas tempers rajas by offering stability and encouraging rest. Rajas lights a fire under your tamasic ass to awaken your passion and get you off that couch.

Sattva (United or Attached)

Balance between tamas and rajas allows sattva to manifest and for your true essence to be illuminated. As Rolf Sovik of the Himalayan Institute wrote in an article for *Yoga International*, "Cultivating sattva—by making choices in life that elevate awareness and foster unselfish joy—is a principal goal of yoga." When you're able to cultivate a sattvic state of mind, you transcend the demands of the ego, enter into a state of pure awareness, and unite in love with the world around you. You may feel a profound sense of connection—a sense that all's right with the world—the way I did that day on Greenwich Avenue. There is no longer any separation between you and others or between your actions and your basic goodness. You serve, not for your own ego or for your personal aggrandizement; you serve because you must. The quality of sattva is clear and balanced; it promotes adaptability, goodness, and living in harmony with nature. *Sat* means truth, the truth that comes from your soul. Sattva is living from that truth, living from love. Pure sattva is being aware without being ensnared. It is looking for—and finding—the good in everyone and in every situation you find yourself in. As Billy says, seeing God in it all.

Being sattvic, however, isn't a one-and-done. You must commit over and over again to actions, thoughts, and habits that promote confidence, clarity, and compassion. Understanding the qualities of each guna can help you get there a little sooner and stay a little longer.

A CALL TO ACTION

My visit to the farm in Uganda opened my eyes to all the ways in which yoga—as permaculture—could make the planet a healthier, more conscious place for all beings. My conversation with Tibyangye opened my eyes to all the ways in which what I was doing was not, in fact, making sattvic choices. I clearly still had work to do. Back home, I began to work with the gunas to better understand my own tendencies. Could I, as Rolf Sovik suggests, begin to see how to temper my rajasic urges, count on tamas to slow things down, and focus on presence and the deep listening sattva encourages?

When we cultivate a more loving presence through a sattvic lifestyle, we vow to be more conscious of how we care for the planet and other species, and how we care for one another and for ourselves. Without love, change is ephemeral; with love, it is everlasting. Without love, we are fractured; with love, we are whole. Serve from love, from the truth of your soul, and regardless of what someone else does or what they believe, you can show up in love. With that love, anything is possible—including peace.

I have long prayed to wake up. I've prayed for peace, and I have prayed to know God. Every challenge I have faced, every lesson I've learned along the path has been an answer to those prayers. The lessons keep coming as the challenges keep presenting themselves—each one more nuanced and complex than the last. And the answers? They are rarely what I expect. But that's what waking up looks like, isn't it? What I do know is this: if you want to be part of the solution and not part of the problem, if you want a society that is equitable and just, or if you want to dismantle the systems that divide instead of unite, you must begin with yourself. Do your inner work. You may need to dismantle the systems *within* first—balancing those fundamental forces yoga calls the gunas over and over again—that keep you from truly committing to justice. And then, as Billy taught, love bigger than you ever thought possible. That's the soul's journey; that's a revolution worth loving for.

THE HEART OF AN ANGEL

11

THERE ARE MOMENTS in life that take your breath away, moments that touch your soul, and moments that break your heart. Little spaces in time that mark shifts in perception and expand your consciousness in unexpected ways. Cambodia was one of those moments for me.

I traveled to Cambodia to visit my friend Scott Neeson, an Australian man who founded the Cambodian Children's Fund (CCF), a nonprofit aid organization in Phnom Penh. We at Off the Mat thought that CCF would be a great organization to support with funding, especially considering that Scott had been a long-time student of yoga. CCF is comprised of five centers, which provide shelter, education, community outreach, and food for around two thousand children, as well as many other services, including a medical center, maternity care, and vocational training.

The organization works to make a dent in the lasting effects of the Pol Pot regime and the unfathomable horrors it had inflicted on the country, including the systematic genocide that killed so many Cambodians less than thirty years before. I was looking forward to learning more about CCF's work and was more committed than ever to practicing service through love after my experience in Uganda.

I arrived in Phnom Penh, a modern city struggling to emerge from the crumbled remnants of a country fractured by war. I dropped my things off at my beautiful hotel, its architecture evidence of the past French colonization, and then jumped into a tuk-tuk—a three-wheeled bicycle-driven cart. After a harrowing ride through the chaotic streets, the driver deposited me at the guarded and gated entrance to CCF. Scott met me at the front door and proceeded to take me from room to room to see the kids at their studies. Some were being instructed in math and English by local educators, some were learning practical skills like sewing, and others were being introduced to their cultural history, traditions, and arts by Cambodian elders who were survivors of the regime. We sat with the kids at lunch, where large trays of rice, chicken, and vegetables were passed around. The room was filled with laughter and chatter as the children clambered for our attention. I noticed several children who were much more subdued, sitting off to the side, away from all the activity. Scott told me that they were new, and it would take them some time to trust and understand their surroundings.

"Where do they all come from?" I asked.

"Why don't we take a drive out there," Scott replied, "so you can see for yourself?"

By "out there" Scott meant Steung Meanchey, the city's garbage dump, where the children lived before coming to CCF. It's important, he told me, to grasp the reality that children all over the world experience, especially when the systems in place are corrupt and the cycle of poverty has been pervasive for generations. He visits the dump every day, he said, because often children are left there to fend for themselves, and if he and his team don't get to them, sex traffickers will.

I jumped at the chance. I wanted to go to Steung Meanchey and see for myself how the staff engaged with the families who live and work there. Because I knew that environments like this could be intense, I normally made a point of doing my sadhana beforehand. I'd take a moment to meditate and pray before walking into any place that could potentially be overwhelming. I'd check in with my body to make sure I could ground and be fully present to what I saw, without judgment, especially when I was in a culture I didn't know or understand.

But not this time. In fact, without much thought at all, I piled into Scott's car feeling confident and excited. After all, I reasoned, I've done this before; I know what to expect, and I can handle anything that comes up. Uh huh. Let's see how that goes.

▼

Bouncing along the streets of Phnom Penh on the way to the dump, Scott tells me more about the Pol Pot regime; the genocide that claimed millions of Cambodian lives; the traumas that remain; and the lack of financial, emotional, and psychological support for the survivors and their descendants. Families were torn apart, he says, communities separated, and the brightest of the bright targeted and murdered. Alcoholism, drug abuse, and sexual and domestic violence were rampant, and many of the systems in place to combat them were ineffective and corrupt.

Scott stops first in a small village just outside of the dump. He wants to show me the medical center the nonprofit had built, which provides free services and care to anyone in the area who needs it. As we walk down the path, a group of village women descend upon us. They are frantic, talking wildly over each other in Khmer. Although I can't understand the language, it's clear that something very, very bad has happened.

I see a small, thin man standing behind the women, slightly off to the side. They keep gesturing at him, and I get that he's the focus of their concern. He, like everyone else who lives on the dump, is filthy, but what catches my attention is a clean, bright-red scarf wound around his neck and hanging down the front of his torso. He has his hand on the scarf, pressing it to his throat. I can't take my eyes off of it, and in the middle of what is clearly an emergency, I find myself wondering, *How, in all this mess, could he have found such a clean scarf? It's so red and bright.* He looks at me, acutely aware that I'm staring at him. I take my attention off the scarf just long enough to meet his eyes. They are filled with tears . . . and something else, though I'm not sure what. He looks down at the ground.

I turn my attention back to the women shouting over each other. I feel like I'm watching this scene play out from afar, even though I am standing smack in the middle of it. I lean in a little closer and can just make out a few words in English as they keep trying to get Scott to understand. I hear "cut," "glass," and "die." Then I hear one of them say "blood."

Blood?

I look over at the man again. Suddenly, I realize the scarf he's holding isn't a scarf, it isn't red, and it's definitely not clean. It's a tattered piece of dirty cloth that he's pressing against his neck; the color comes from the blood pouring from his throat. I look again and see there's also blood on his shirt, on his arms, and on the ground in front of him. How had I missed that?

Shocked and alarmed, I look to Scott for an explanation, as we lead the man to the medical center for immediate care. Scott quietly explains that the man tried to kill himself, only moments before, by slicing his neck open with a piece of broken glass. It didn't quite work. The women found him and dragged him out to get help.

Afterward, Scott tells me suicide goes against their belief in the sacredness of all living beings. However, this man will suffer even more for staying alive because he has brought shame to himself and his whole family. I now know what else I saw in his eyes.

We get back in Scott's car and drive silently over to the dump. I feel shaky and am having trouble grounding my energy. I remind myself to breathe and self-regulate. I close my eyes and try to focus on my feet. I can't. All I can see is the image of the man holding his throat. Blood that I couldn't see as blood, gushing from a wound I couldn't see as a wound. I open my eyes and stare at the literal mountain of garbage in front of me. I've seen a lot in my travels, but nothing like this.

We park at the foot of the dump, and Scott leads me around the periphery where homes, linked side by side, are held together with corrugated metal, random pieces of wood, cardboard, Styrofoam, and any other found objects. Floors are made of dirt or planks of loose wood, no one has water or electricity, bathrooms are nonexistent, and the air is toxic. Everywhere I look men, women, and children are going about their lives—some stretched out on makeshift cots, others playing or working, and many engaged in conversation with their neighbors. To get from one place to another, we walk through a network of narrow, muddy, waste-strewn alleyways. I keep covering my mouth and nose because the pervasive smell of sewage and refuse is making me nauseous. And why the hell am I wearing flip-flops? Every time I take a step, wet, contaminated crud oozes over the sides, covering my bare feet in filth.

I see people in their homes lying together in heaps, limb over limb, brushing away flies and trying to stay out of the hot sun. I see women squatting on the ground in groups, counting beans or cooking rice over an open fire. All around me, babies are crying, and mothers are trying to soothe them by placing the end of a water-soaked cloth in their mouths to suck on. Haunted and desperate, small children with hair the color of rust from lack of iron, eyes watery and infected, teeth black and rotten, gesture toward me, begging for food. Their bellies extend over stick-thin legs, a sure indication of malnutrition. I see countless scars, bruises, and cuts, signs of living on the dump and of the abuse that comes from traumatized and angry parents with too many children and not enough food to feed them.

Each time I look in their direction, the children look away. Not once, as we wander through their homes, do I see a child smile. I struggle to reconcile the children here with the bright and energetic kids I met at CCF. Why are so many still here? Why haven't they gone to CCF? Don't they want to?

I can't imagine why anyone would choose to come here when they have a clean bed and ample food and water at CCF; on the other hand, this is their home, I remind myself, this is where their families are, and there's a certain level of comfort in that. For children to come to CCF, their families (parents, parent, or guardian) must give permission. Once they do that, it's understood that they can see their children anytime they wish. Of course, CCF also houses many children who have been abandoned by families who couldn't afford to keep them. These children are among the most vulnerable because sex traffickers often patrol the dump looking for kids who appear to be alone and unprotected.

I understand that the children at CCF have a chance at creating a long, more healthful, and successful life for themselves, but what about all these other children I see here? Children whose families don't want to let them go, children as young as two who climb through the garbage, scavenging for metal and plastic to sell so their families can survive. Don't they deserve a shot at happiness too? Of course they do. I feel a lump in my throat as my sadness for these families grows, along with my anger at the system that keeps them oppressed.

I follow Scott back to the truck and begin handing out the food that we've brought. From overstuffed boxes, I pull out a small bottle of soymilk, some rice, and packaged soup. The children rush toward us from all directions; Scott smiles brightly, completely unfazed by the onslaught. I get pushed back against the truck and look out into the crowd that has swelled to what feels like at least a hundred people. Holy shit. Where did they all come from? Small hands tug at my clothes and grab at my hair, desperate for food and attention. I hand out what's in the truck, but quickly realize that we've only brought enough to feed a third of the people gathered. My heart breaks. How do I decide who gets to eat? Do I pick the starving six-year-old with his little brother in tow, or the pregnant mother carrying an infant in her arms, or the toothless old man whose legs can barely hold him up? Why didn't we bring more? Is this it for the week? What about tomorrow? I can't bear to choose, and I can't bear to look at the people around me. Staring straight ahead, I hand out the remainder of the food and milk randomly without making eye contact.

Once we finish distributing everything, Scott leads me to a small, isolated shack set slightly apart from the others. There are no doors or windows, just three makeshift walls holding up a plastic roof and a blue tarp the family can pull down before they sleep to cover the opening. For now it's peeled back to expose the inside of the shack, which is mostly empty. Lying on the ground, a woman in the last stages of her pregnancy, naked from the waist up, has her legs spread apart. Her head is bandaged, and blood seeps through the soiled cloth. As we approach, she makes a feeble attempt to cover herself, but she is too weak. Squatting close by, a little girl tends to her mother's head wound. As soon as she sees Scott, she leans forward and covers her mother's breasts with a rag, sparing her the indignity she knows her mother feels.

The woman's husband sits on a wooden box nearby. He attempts to gets up when he sees Scott walk in, but stumbles and falls. Scott tells me that the husband, a violent alcoholic, often beats his wife and children; the woman's bandages hide the effects of a blow he gave her with a hammer. They have had twelve children, seven of whom have died. The little girl, Shrey Heng, is the oldest—Scott thinks she might be about nine—and must care for her mother and her siblings because her mother can no longer work. Her father doesn't work either and spends whatever money they can scrounge on booze.

Scott wants the father to allow Shrey Heng and her siblings to come to CCF, but he refuses. How will they get money, he wants to know? The last time they talked, the father offered to sell Shrey Heng to Scott, which is illegal. The father couldn't care less—he believes it will benefit the family in the long run. Scott's fear, of course, is that someone else will be more than willing to buy Shrey Heng and that she could easily be sold into sexual slavery for the rest of her life. Scott has appealed to the father on many occasions, to no avail. For whatever reason, Scott is hoping my presence will somehow make a difference; that the man might agree to let Shrey Heng leave with us that day, which is what her mother had wanted for a long time.

I approach Shrey Heng and squat down low so we are eye to eye. I tell her my name. She says nothing but continues to look at my face. She has dark circles under her eyes, and she is caked with dirt and mud from head to toe. Her knees are pulled into her chest; her shoulders slump forward. I want so badly to hug her, to tell her everything will be okay, but it's not my place. And, anyway, I'm not convinced that those words will ever be true.

"Hey," I say smiling, hoping to make a connection, "you have a scar like I do!" I point at the small scar that cuts through my right eyebrow, the result of a minor accident when I was an infant, and then at the one that cuts through hers. "*Dauchaknea, dauchaknea,* same, same," I say, remembering the phrase I saw on some T-shirts in Siem Reap. She stares at my eyebrow and shakes her head. "Dauchaknea, dauchaknea," she says quietly. I immediately realize how wrong I was *and* how correct I was. "Dauchaknea, dauchaknea" literally means "same, same—*but different.*" Yes, she has a scar, and so do I, but the similarity ends there. Looking more closely, I notice fresh blood seeping from hers, as well as the other scars and open wounds on her face, results of the terrible beatings she has endured her whole life. There is nothing "same, same" about it.

She turns away from me and begins to rub her mother's feet, making soft, cooing sounds of comfort. I feel foolish. I turn and watch Scott face the father; they're both waving their arms in front of each other and shouting in Khmer. Scott catches my eye and gestures for me to come over. I walk toward them, and the smell of alcohol mixed with strong body odor makes me once again clap my hand over my nose. I can't help but imagine him beating his wife and children right here in this very room, and the thought infuriates me. My revulsion makes it impossible for me to meet his eyes; my anger prevents me from uttering a word. Scott keeps trying to get me to engage, but I can only stare at the ground. The father once again refuses Scott's plea for permission to take his children to CCF. Defeated, we walk away. As we leave the shack, I glance back toward Shrey Heng, but she's too busy tending to her mother to pay us any mind. I know I have failed her.

Scott is discouraged but not about to give up. He vows to continue trying until those kids are safe. Now it's time to see if there are "new" children in the dump he's not aware of; children who may have been abandoned during the night. Scott snatches some thick rubber boots from the truck and instructs me to put them on. I'm relieved but can't help wondering why I didn't put them on in the first place. My feet are coated with sewage and who knows what else, all the way up to my ankles. I wipe them down with some discarded newspaper, put on the boots, and off we go, deeper into the thick of it, with a bevy of children tagging along. We walk on thousands of tons of paper, clothes, broken glass, needles, rancid food, toxic waste, and shit, relying on the children to make sure we stay on the safest pathways. The children are mostly barefoot or have on a single flip-flop or shoe; filthy rags, substituting as bandages, cover their bleeding feet.

Often a child takes my hand and guides me so I don't step on a sinkhole and get sucked under. These things are everywhere, and it's not unusual for children to fall in and drown in the waste and debris. Besides death-by-sinkholes, Scott tells me, there's the danger of being run over by one of the enormous dump trucks that barrel through the area or succumbing to dehydration, infections, exposure, disease, or malnutrition. I can't bear it. I want to take them away from this place. I want them safe. Instead, I follow helplessly as they make certain that we remain safe while we navigate the trash heap that is their home.

After a while, we come upon a woman digging furiously through the trash, looking for anything recyclable that she can sell. Holding a small, ragged plastic bag, a little girl also searches for anything of value. As the woman sees us approaching, she glances furtively in all directions. Suddenly, she leaps up, grabs hold of the young child and literally tosses her in our direction, yelling "Chaul tow! Chaul tow! Chaul tow!"—Go! Go! Go! She obviously knows who Scott is; she wants him to take her child away quickly. Scott moves toward her, speaking gently in Khmer, as he shakes his head and hands her back her child, whose name is Navy. The mother is crying. Scott explains to me that, when she saw her husband wasn't nearby, she seized the moment to save her child. Sadly, it's not possible for him to take a child without both parents' consent. "*Suam chaul tow . . .*" she pleads—Please go, please go—as she pushes Navy closer to us. We indicate, again, that we are so sorry, and turn away. I look back at the woman crouched on the ground, still crying, and hugging her child tightly to her chest.

We continue walking; the scorching midday sun intensifies the stench of the massive field of garbage we are now standing in. Little ones dig into piles of fresh trash, recently dumped by large trucks, for any treasure that might bring value. As soon as they see us coming, they gesture for water and food. I look over at Scott, but he's already kneeling down, cleaning out a little girl's foot wound, smiling and chatting with her as he applies a fresh bandage.

I turn back to the children now surrounding me; we are all covered with flies. I swat the buzzing insects and then cover my nose and mouth to block the overwhelming stink of rancid decay. I know I should be engaging with them. But honestly, I just want out. I want to leave so badly and go back to my beautiful, clean hotel. I want to call my boyfriend and tell him about this horror. I want to take a bath. I want to be anywhere other than here. My mind and body struggle to stay put, to remain present, but I feel myself disconnecting. I am sad and angry. Life here is unfair. These kids are fucked. Their families are fucked. Their culture is fucked. The whole system is fucked. I realize that I'm starting to spin out, just like I did after my first day at the children's shelter in LA, but I feel powerless to stop. I think about the corrupt Cambodian government, the US government, and the incomprehensible slaughter that led to the circumstances I am witnessing. My mind continues on to rail against the genocide happening in Darfur and how history is repeating itself and how the global community isn't doing enough to stop it. My thoughts move on to the extermination of more than 6 million Jews, gay people, Roma, people of color, and people with disabilities before and during World War II. To the abused sex workers I met in India and the countless number of children I have met in South Africa and Uganda who were dying of AIDS. To the teenagers I taught at the shelter, kids who wear engagement rings from their pimps as a sign of their "commitment." To Shrey Heng. Will she ever know joy? Will any of them?

And then, finally, my thoughts turn to God, and rage rises up from the pit of my soul. What is going on here? Why do some people have so much and others so little? Why do pain and suffering exist like this if we are "all One"? How could Billy believe that we're all here to learn what love is when so many are here to learn what survival is—one fucking day at a time? *Show me evidence of that love in this horrific place,* I think to myself. *Where the fuck is God?*

Just then I feel a small hand in mine. I look down and see a young boy peering up at me. He's covered in dirt, and his head's wrapped in mud-soaked rags to protect him from the sweltering sun. We stare at each other, and I wait for him to ask for water, or food, or safe passage out of this place. He says nothing. He just holds my hand and studies my face. We remain like that for a moment, and then he smiles. It's the first time I've seen a child smile at Steung Meanchey. I smile back. He nods his head slightly, squeezes my hand, turns around, and walks away.

A moment later, I realize he's left something in my hand. I open it to see what it could be.

In the center of my palm lies a small mound of hardened dirt. I break the soil apart to find within a silver and red medallion, shaped like a heart, which catches the light of the noonday sun. I stare at it for a moment. All the pent-up emotions from that day rise up and make themselves known. I take a breath, the first true, deep inhale of the day. As I exhale, I can feel the tension I have been holding melt from my body and soften my heart. I lower my head and cry.

I think once again of Billy. "And what is this love we awaken to?" he'd asked. "It's God, Seane. It's inside of us, and it's what connects us to one another. Fully." *Of course*, I think, *of course*. "See the soul," he said, "and you will understand what unites us all." Love. That is what unites us, that is who we are. That is God. This little angel has shown me that God *is* here. God is everywhere, and most certainly all over that garbage dump, but, once again, not so apparent within me. I forgot to ignore the story. I forgot to see the soul. And when I did, I also forgot to love. God may be everywhere, but if my heart is shut down, I can't see God. If my heart is shut down, I can only do harm. Without love, without God, I am the problem.

I look back down at the heart, and it occurs to me that Tibyangye was right. I may have brought the food and money, but without the love, *I am* disordered. *I am* out of harmony. *I am* in the way. And, even with the best of intentions, until I understand that, I will only continue to create harm. That is what he meant. Jesus, it's just the same friggin' lesson, over and over. Will I ever get it? Damn. I have so much to learn.

Why are you here, Seane? I hear Tibyangye's voice in my head.

I look again for the little boy. He's nowhere to be found. I silently thank him, then turn my face up toward the sky, close my eyes, and will myself to pray. "Why *am* I here?" I ask, and in a flash the answer comes, "To love bigger than I ever thought was possible, myself, each other, this planet, and God as One." I say this over and over. Like a mantra. May it plant seeds in my soul . . . may it fill the hole in my heart.

Clutching the medallion, I look around me. The trucks still move forward and back, the children continue to work tirelessly. The garbage, the stench, and the oppression remain, of course. Nothing has changed—except me. The little boy's gift, a symbol of his own heart, was like a bolt of lightning that jolted me awake. My judgments and my own pain hadn't allowed me to see the individual souls buried deep in the muck of their own lives and to understand the individual, cultural, and ancestral stories that had held them captive for so long. His little heart broke mine wide open so that I could *feel* the suffering of others. I finally understood. My dharma, my spiritual practice, is to be of service, to do whatever

I can to ease suffering, without any thought of what's in it for me. However, unless and until I can remain fully in the present and see the truth of what is—not what I judge it to be—unless and until I can show up only from love, as Tibyangye taught me, I'll just be in the way. I had most certainly been in the way. But that little boy's gesture gave me a second chance. So who is serving whom?

Scott and I backtrack through the dump to find the fathers of Shrey Heng and Navy. At first, they're belligerent and resistant, but this time I'm ready to listen and try to understand their concerns. I breathe and make eye contact, and feel into their pain, even as I silently acknowledge that these men embody a level of trauma and suffering I cannot possibly comprehend. No one ever said understanding meant condoning, but for some reason I've been afraid it might. But now, it makes sense. When I can commit to seeing them as individuals, I can meet, with humility, the power of Spirit that resides within each man. Perhaps they could see Spirit in me, as well, because Shrey Heng and Navy leave with us that night.

I continue to work with Scott at the dump, engaging with the children and their families. As time goes on, I'm able to focus less on the despair and more on the remarkable resilience and resourcefulness present all around me. By doing so, I now see the smiles I failed to see earlier; I feel the connection between siblings, the tenderness mothers wrap their babies in, the ways in which children and adults learn not only how to survive but how to live. But let's get real. Never once do I gloss over or fail to see the conditions and the pain these people endure. Their lives, their situation, are truly horrific. But, when I replace pity with compassion, I see that change can happen; change, in fact, *is* happening, and healing *is* possible.

With change comes possibility; with possibility we find hope; out of hope springs action. And action, fueled by love and knowledge, gives rise to authentic service. Authentic and compassionate service can create true and everlasting peace and help bring about a world that is fair, free, and just.

TEACHINGS FROM CAMBODIA
PRIVILEGE, HUMILITY, AND GRACE

By the time I got to Cambodia, I had more awareness around conscious service, but only slightly. What Tibyangye said had really stuck with me. I didn't come with my checkbook in hand and a list of powerful connections, like I did when I went to Uganda. I didn't come with a prescription for healthy action that I planned to impose on others, like I had done at the shelter in LA. I wanted to "commit to love," as Tibyangye had taught me, and so I showed up ready to be put to work doing whatever the community asked of me. If they wanted me to paint a fence, plant a garden, or fund a project, then that's what I'd do. I would take their lead, listen more than talk, and make certain that I kept my privilege in check. Unfortunately, it didn't quite go that way. Because the work just never ends, my desire to show up in love, instead of *being* love, coupled with my rajastic, Tigger-like enthusiasm, wasn't enough. There were plenty of obstacles that stood in my way even though I had spent what felt like a lifetime doing my inner work in order to live my dharma authentically. As Mona told me the day we met, "What gets in the way *is* the way."

My experience in Cambodia was a reminder that doing the inner work Mona encouraged me to do is absolutely essential in order to be fully present. But it also taught me that I must do the outer work necessary to understand what I'm being present to. I hadn't taken the time to learn and understand the history, the culture, or the needs of the people I showed up to serve. I hadn't considered the complexities of the systems designed to oppress and my role within them, or how deep my privilege ran. I hadn't counted on the ways I would project my perceptions onto a culture and its people that I wasn't a part of and didn't truly comprehend. I came with the intention of serving from love, but I couldn't actually do that until I overcame my ignorance, my ego, and the other obstacles that stood in my way.

THE FIVE OBSTACLES

According to the yoga tradition, certain mental and emotional roadblocks interfere with our ability to connect, to see the truth, and to serve. These *kleshas*, or personal obstacles, include ignorance (*avidya*), pride or ego (*asmita*), desire (*raga*), aversion (*dvesha*), and fear or attachment (*abhinivesa*). Yoga doesn't really see any of these as character flaws (thank God); they're more like interruptions or disturbances that throw us off track. And it's part of our asana and meditation practice to identify and work with them. You'll notice that these kleshas start with our mental obstacles and then move into our emotional ones. Every one of these obstacles demonstrates how privilege can get in the way of authentic service, especially when a person isn't aware of their privilege.

Ignorance (Avidya)

Ignorance, first and foremost, is mistaking the small self for our Highest Self, the ego for the soul. Avidya doesn't refer to being stupid or clueless; it simply means "not knowing." It implies that we don't know what we don't know, that we act from our limiting beliefs as though they're universal truths. Avidya is pretty much the root of all the other kleshas; it's the biggest barrier to connecting with others because in our ignorance, we fail to distinguish our soul's truth from our ego's interference. Ignorance causes us to contract around our limiting beliefs. At the shelter, at the permaculture farm, and finally at Steung Meanchey, I failed to see what was right in front of me because I was looking through a distorted lens. As a result, my ego was fixated on what I was capable or incapable of doing *for* those in front of me instead of actually being present *with* them. I was so busy projecting my own understanding of what the people I witnessed lacked—and what I thought they needed—that I failed to learn, listen, and feel into our shared humanity. As a result, I failed to serve from love.

We must do our homework first—on a personal as well as a global level—if we wish to be of real service. Before we go into a new situation, the onus is on us to understand what we're going into. Before we visit a new country or culture, like I did, we need to become familiar with its customs, beliefs, cultural differences, and traditions. We need to approach the experience with an awareness of how our own perspective differs from that of the people we are about to meet and a willingness to let go of the truths, values, and opinions that we bring with us, which reflect only our own life experience and cultural reality, not objective facts. But so often, we don't. Ignorance is an insidious byproduct of privilege, a subconscious refusal to acknowledge or become aware of things that make us feel uncomfortable or guilty. Privilege gives us the ability to live our lives unaware of things that other people have to struggle with every day. For example, the privilege of being born a US citizen could mean being ignorant of the daily fear experienced by those without proper documentation, and the privilege of having no disabilities or health conditions could mean being ignorant of how much time and resources it takes to navigate health and insurance systems when you do.

Ignorance often comes from fear, and fear keeps us from moving out of ignorance. Our nervous system is hardwired to fear anything we don't understand, which can be critical for our survival. Fortunately, as beings with souls, we have the ability to move beyond our hardwiring, to seek out connection and undermine ignorance, which will then eradicate fear. Our fear keeps others at a safe distance, and as long as we close our ears to the wisdom of others, we will remain there. As long as we see only with our eyes and fail to witness from Divine Consciousness, we will continue to confuse the ego with the soul. And, remember, the ego rejects the unknown, clinging desperately to the known. The soul craves experience and opens to whatever presents itself.

Going into any situation that's unfamiliar to you, it's important to take the time to assess and then ground your energy. Asana is an important part of that process; it allows you to feel your feet underneath you and creates a firm, physical foundation so you don't lose your balance, literally or figuratively. Pranayama, meditation, and prayer can all help center you and regulate your nervous system. I know when I don't do any of that, I can't think clearly, and I react or shut down out of fear. That's what happened almost immediately at Steung Meanchey. How else could I have failed to see that the "clean, red scarf" around a man's neck was, in fact, a dirty rag he had pressed against his throat to stanch the flow of blood from a self-inflicted wound? Conscious breathing and a moment of prayer before I jumped in Scott's truck would have helped stabilize my mind and keep me present. Asking more questions of Scott, instead of coming across as if I knew what I was doing, would have helped me prepare as well and lessen my fear. I didn't do any of that. I was at my edge, and none of my tools were working. Why? Because I forgot to use them!

Pride (Asmita)

Pride is what B.K.S. Iyengar called the "insanity of individualism, when it should be the joy of singularity." Individualism causes us to despise differences and create separation; singularity allows us to embrace the uniqueness of each soul and find joy in our differences. Individualism feasts on the Western hierarchy of who's more worthy, whose traits are more valuable. And judgment serves that hierarchy: I am industrious, you are lazy. I am right, you are mistaken. I am whole, you are broken. You need fixing, I can fix you. Pride allows us to create harm and separation by "otherizing" instead of unifying. We lead with judgment

and not with openness. My pride created a false sense of security, which convinced me "I got this; I'll be fine." I wasn't.

Pride puts and keeps blinders on. In Uganda, I participated in an unequal power dynamic because I tried to impose my solutions onto what I saw as the problems of the people I met—when in fact no one had asked me to, nor could I fully comprehend the complexities of their situation. Power-over is dominance, whether we are conscious of our actions or not. Power-under is always oppression. Those wielding power set up a dynamic in which they can take center stage. Everything is all about them, they are the heroes of every story, and only they can ensure that the story ends happily ever after—at least *their* version of that.

In Cambodia, my pride and unexamined advantage also kept me separate, but in a different way. This time, it prevented me from connecting and serving because I couldn't fathom the suffering, the filth, and the despair—it didn't make sense to me. Why didn't more children just leave the dump and go to the warmth and security of CCF? I certainly would have sent *my* kids to CCF in a New

York minute if it were available. And no way would I have stayed with someone who beat my kids—or me. What was wrong with these people? Didn't parents want their kids to be safe and well cared for? I didn't understand, and therefore, I judged them harshly. They didn't perform like I thought they should—especially the men. In my fear, anger, and helplessness, I failed to grasp the full impact of the ancestral and cultural trauma playing out in front of me or the systems in place that perpetuate the suffering. I took note of my own coping mechanisms (dissociation) but inwardly railed against theirs (alcohol, aggression, detachment, sleep). I named my own triggers but couldn't make room for theirs.

Desire (Raga)

Desire is not always an affliction. Desire can get us off our asses and drive us to act. If we want to "serve and see the world as whole," Eknath Easwaran says, "we have to first shed the ego, and let go of what keeps us separate." In the words of my friend Teo Drake, "We've got to have skin in the game." Raga becomes an obstacle when we get attached to the pleasures and rewards of our actions, when we serve solely to elevate our image or our own self-worth. My insistence in Uganda that I knew best how to alleviate suffering was ego-driven and, therefore, not sustainable. I wanted to be seen as competent and indispensable as well as compassionate and connected. In Cambodia, however, my desire was a bit more complex. I couldn't bear the filth, the suffering, the palpable violence all around me. I wanted to address the root causes of their suffering, absolutely, even though I hadn't a clue how. But I also have to admit that I wanted desperately to alleviate my own discomfort. The first desire represents a heartfelt longing to serve; the second one presents an obstacle to that service. Eventually, thanks to the deep soul service offered by the young boy and his heart, I vowed to stay present, let myself see a bigger spiritual picture and my part in it, and do whatever was possible to not cause additional suffering.

Aversion (Dvesha)

Aversion is an emotional response that causes us to judge something or someone we don't understand as repulsive, hateful, or just plain wrong. Like raga, dvesha is not, in and of itself, an affliction. It allows us to notice injustice, hateful behaviors, and oppressive actions that cause suffering—and commit to righting those wrongs. But it becomes an obstacle when we equate behaviors and actions with the people doing them—and fail to see the circumstances surrounding all that. I had a harder time with aversion in Steung Meanchey than in Uganda. In Uganda, I could *see* the tangible results of the organization's mission, the effects their efforts had on the children they served. In Cambodia, when Scott showed me around CCF, I immediately saw what they created and how it had made a difference in the children's lives. Both of these organizations made sense to my Western conditioning. It was neat and tidy. I was exposed to the solution, not so much the suffering. But when I foolishly rushed in to "serve" the people at the dump, without properly preparing intellectually, emotionally, or physically, I recoiled in disgust and wanted to bolt. When Scott tried to educate me, I heard his words and understood them on a superficial level, but there was no way I could experience their full impact without being, quite literally, in the mud and the blood and the pain.

When I was at Steung Meanchey, I witnessed a level of violence and abuse that shook me to my core. How *dare* that father beat his wife and kids? How *dare* he work his wife to the bone just so he could get wasted? I was so repulsed I couldn't even look directly at him. My aversion ran so deep that I couldn't see God in the details and refused to even entertain the idea that this man's true essence—masked by years of suffering—was the same as mine, the same as everyone else's. I failed to consider what brought him to his pain, to drugs and alcohol. I refused to see that the only outlet for his suffering was to recreate what he felt in others. The oppressed becomes the oppressor. Finally, my aversion prevented me from engaging compassionately. I, too, became the oppressor when my judgments did not allow me to ignore the story and see the divinity in this tortured man's soul. My aversion and my judgments prevented me from serving or from connecting with anyone.

Fear and Attachment (Abhinivesha)

Fear and attachment are what keep us clinging to what we know and who we think we are—our desires and even our aversions. Abhinivesha is a manifestation of our ego, which fights to the death to stay alive. And, of course, it also comes out of ignorance and adversely affects our ability to think, act, and connect with clarity or compassion. Fear destabilizes the nervous system. We already know that when we're stressed, we don't think clearly; we react, overreact, or even shut down. I'm definitely quicker to judge when I'm in my ego. Our need to cling to our small self and all its outward manifestations—pride, wealth, possessions, privilege—arises out of fear.

Abhinivesha for me, as a person with privilege, is about attachment to being seen as a good person, a compassionate person. My ego is far more likely to show up as a would-be savior, like it did in Uganda, than as a hideous troll. But this attachment gets in the way of really examining systems of oppression and my culpability in them. If I'm more attached to my self-identity as a good person than I am driven by a desire to end suffering,

that's an obstacle. If someone points out a way in which my actions are causing harm or participating in oppression, and my first thought is "I can't possibly be causing harm because I'm such a good person," that's abhinivesha. I have to be willing to sacrifice my image of myself as a good person in order to be a whole person who has both faults and graces.

▼

Any one of these afflictions increases separation. Privilege is what allows any of us to choose when to serve and when to walk away if things get too hot to handle—it allows us to erect barriers so we don't *have to* see or feel things that cause us to feel guilty, afraid, or powerless. Metaphorically, it's like discovering black mold on your walls and deciding to paint or paper over it instead of getting rid of it or figuring out what caused it in the first place. At Steung Meanchey, there were several times I wanted to get the hell out of there, go back to my hotel, and put the day behind me—call my boyfriend and whine, watch a movie, take a soothing bath, or order room service. Shrey Heng and others at the dump had no choice but to remain in their struggles and do whatever they could to survive. My privilege gave me the freedom to choose. I didn't earn this freedom; I was born into it—the luck of the draw. But if I really believe we are all One and there's no separation, like yoga has taught me, then running away would mean that I'd be abandoning me, my highest Self, and my dharma—my true purpose for being. I chose to stay.

HOW ARE WE ALL ONE?

Bearing witness to such suffering in India, Uganda, and Cambodia—as well as in my own country—woke me up to the hypocrisy of the way the yoga concept "we are all One" gets used and understood in Western, predominantly white yoga contexts. At its core, yoga teaches that all life is interconnected; "we are all One" speaks to this spiritual truth. Yet this phrase often gets used in ways that ignore this essence. "We are all One" doesn't mean that we are all the same. It means that when one being suffers, all beings suffer; when one group over-consumes, another group goes hungry.

When I eagerly tried to make a connection with Shrey Heng because of our matching scars, I was ignoring the huge differences between us that were right in front of my eyes. Seeing and naming differences is not what causes division or inequality—and ignoring differences is definitely not the way to heal injustice. Living from the truth that we all are One means acknowledging that, as physics teaches, every action has an equal and opposite reaction—both on a molecular level and a global one. It means committing to doing the work necessary to decrease the suffering and violence that exists and taking accountability for our role in that suffering.

Often our ignorance or pride can keep us from understanding how our actions and inactions, privileges and biases fracture connection and cause suffering. It's tempting to want to benefit from the sentiment of "we are all One" without having to face the painful flip side: our complicity in inequity. But interconnectedness teaches that if I am advantaged by a system, my advantage comes at the cost of someone else being disadvantaged—and the only cure is to undo my advantage; that's the only way to break down the separation between me and other beings. If we harken back to what Tibyangye explained about permaculture, it all makes sense. It's all about balance. When one part gets more than it needs, the whole is compromised. When one group of people takes more than its share of the earth's resources, others are left with less than they need. Eventually, everyone suffers. "Same, same but different" means we see the differences, acknowledge the inequities that exist, and work to change the systemic power dynamics that create them.

When we commit to a spiritual practice, like yoga or meditation or prayer, we experience the Oneness; judgments, impatience, and misunderstandings often fall away. When I initially went to the shelter, I came as someone who had all the answers and, as a result, drove a wedge between me and the young people there. Once I brought them into my practice and into my prayers, I got the connection. I felt into their suffering, as I felt into my own, and found within me ways in which I could participate in their healing and tend to mine as well. When I could do that, there was no longer any separation between us. We were bound by something greater than even our shared humanity. We were bound by compassion and love. We are bound by God.

In Cambodia, an act of pure love from a sweet young boy snapped me out of my ego, woke me up, and deposited me fully conscious in the present moment. Suddenly, I was able to see into the filth, the poverty, the oppression, and the abuse and also feel the love that existed. Food and services were needed, absolutely. That's a given. But without love and without working to understand the role I—and my people—played in the injustice before me, I was just placing one more Band-Aid on a wound. It's not sustainable. I was in Steung Meanchey to understand what it meant to love each other as One, to witness each other, to dignify each other, to hold each other sacred, and to recognize the Self as the same in all beings—even as I acknowledged our differences. That is what yoga means by We Are All One.

We all have our Cambodias—those times where we show up unprepared and we get overwhelmed. But we do the best we can with the tools we have. Each experience allows us to put our yoga into action and identify the obstacles that prevent us from committing to our dharma. And make no mistake: we all have obstacles, or kleshas, to overcome—because of our upbringing, our education, our biases, and even our ancestry. Having obstacles is not the problem; ignoring them and allowing them to cause harm is. So, it's on us to see them, own them, and commit to changing them. This is yoga. This is radical accountability—and radical accountability is a revolutionary act of love.

We serve because we *are* all One. We are all embodied Spirit. We serve because we must—not in order to be the hero or to stockpile good karma and erase the effects of the bad things we've done. We serve because our liberation—and the liberation of all souls—depends on it. We cannot be truly free, we cannot be fully happy, as long as there is suffering in the world. Coming together in love, united in truth, is the only way in which to authentically serve, and it is the only sustainable reason why we should ever feed a body, cure a disease, end a war, touch a hand, or guide a soul.

THE FOUR IMMEASURABLES

Showing up from love is not a form of spiritual bypass; it's not declaring "our thoughts and prayers are with you" in a knee-jerk, bullshit kind of way. Lives are at stake, shit needs to get done, and it needs to get done now. In the presence of suffering, no doubt you'll feel devastated. That's okay. Feel all the feelings, express and release all your rage—and act anyway. Serve anyway. But remember, for service to be truly sustainable, you must choose love over fear and most certainly empathy over sympathy or pity every single time.

Serving from love, keeping love at the forefront of all that we do, means keeping the ego in check, which is a challenging and yet integral part of yoga in action. It is how we can hold ourselves accountable for the ways in which we, consciously or unconsciously, contribute to the suffering of others through our choices, actions, and words. There's a Sanskrit mantra many people often recite during yoga class: *Lokah samastah sukhino bhavantu*, which means "May all beings everywhere be happy and free, and may the thoughts, words, and actions of my own life contribute to that happiness and to that freedom for all."

Reciting mantra and praying are powerful, of course, but in order for real change to happen, we must move those intentions into action. One way to do that is to practice the Four Immeasurables (or *Brahma-viharas*)—friendliness, compassion, empathetic joy, and equanimity—which form the basis of the mantra, as well as the popular loving-kindness meditation.

Here's the thing, though. It's not enough to pray for happiness or wish for an end to suffering. Those are lovely heart-tugging sentiments, but they won't get the job done. We must work to find the *causes* of happiness and alleviate the causes of suffering—for *everyone*, even those we don't understand, even those we believe are evil. This takes engaging the mind as well as expanding the heart. In an article for *Tricycle* magazine, Thai monk Thanissaro Bhikkhu wrote that your heart is the part of your mind that wants everyone to be happy. The head is the part of your mind that has to figure out how to make that happen. Your head and heart have to learn how to

cooperate, he says, so that once your head finds the causes of happiness, your heart can "learn to embrace those causes."

Friendliness (Maitri or Metta)

Some teachers call this goodwill or loving-kindness, but basically *maitri* or *metta* is our wish that everyone find true happiness and the causes of happiness. I sometimes think of metta as a gentle sprinkling of goodwill that we offer to everyone because, let's face it, whether we love them, hate them, or fear them, everyone wants to be happy. And, when our hearts feel particularly open, we can admit that everyone *deserves* that happiness.

Compassion (Karuna)

Remember, compassion means "feeling *with*" or even "suffering with"; it's an earnest desire to alleviate suffering and the causes of suffering—wherever you find them. Indeed, it is what prevents us from turning away from injustice and misery; it reminds us that when one person suffers, we all suffer. Compassion doesn't mean feeling sorry for someone's plight or stepping in to fix or save anyone. If we truly want to alleviate suffering, we must help tear down systems that foster oppression and inequality and build those that support freedom and inclusiveness. Even more, we must each understand how we contribute to those systems—consciously or unconsciously. That's the lesson I had to learn and relearn and learn again—at the children's shelter, in Uganda, and in Cambodia. That's the lesson I will continue to learn.

Empathetic Joy (Mudita)

Another translation for *mudita* is "appreciative joy"—our ability to feel happiness for the good fortune of others. We want others to be happy, right? So, it logically follows that we would rejoice in that happiness. But what if someone's happiness makes no sense to you? Can you love what they love anyway? Can you feel happy for someone who has found joy traveling a path that you would never in a million years choose for yourself? That's mudita. Practicing empathetic joy also means remembering the joy that comes from being alive, from doing your dharma, from connecting with another being,

soul-to-soul. In Cambodia, I needed to remember the joy that comes from simply being present before I could see the joy hidden behind the suffering of the people at the dump. I needed to stop assuming that they could never experience joy or connection or love because of the conditions they faced.

Equanimity (Upeksha or Upekkha)

All four of the immeasurables, according to Buddhism, arise from our essential nature. We are naturally predisposed to want all beings to be happy, to do what we can to alleviate suffering, and to rejoice in the happiness of others. The fourth immeasurable, equanimity, is a bit different. Equanimity is often translated as "standing in the middle," "seeing with patience," or even "looking over," all of which suggest that we see what's in front of us without getting caught by it—without judging it, fearing it, or jumping in to try to fix it. Thanissaro Bhikkhu says that by practicing equanimity, you can see whether you are contributing to or alleviating suffering. He says that when you encounter suffering that you can't stop no matter how hard you try, equanimity prevents you from creating more. Equanimity helps you "channel your energies to areas where you *can* be of help," he says. It also implies "seeing equally," or understanding that your happiness is inseparable from the happiness of others, and your liberation is intimately tied to the liberation of all beings.

The truth is you won't be able to serve everywhere, and you won't be able to alleviate all of the suffering you encounter. None of us will. But you can practice equanimity by connecting inward first in order to minimize the chance of creating more suffering. That is why you get on the mat and breathe. Then you get off the mat, and from that centered place, do whatever it is that needs to be done in order to create peace.

▼

Offering the Brahma-viharas to yourself allows you to discover, in a powerful and loving way, how best you can be of service. These immeasurables allow you to see how your traumas—personal, ancestral, and cultural—and your unprocessed emotions prevent you from being loving, compassionate, and joyful; how your unchecked privileges and inherent biases stop you from learning about and understanding the personal, ancestral, and cultural traumas of those you wish to serve; and finally, how all of that contributes to the suffering of others. By being tender, loving, and ruthlessly honest, we can all begin to heal the fractured places within us, love who we are, and embrace the path toward wholeness we've chosen. Once that happens, we can cast off the veil of ignorance that clouds our ability to see and embrace the humanity in all souls. We can then feel another's pain and also connect with their joy and their Spirit. When we love bigger than we ever imagined possible and embrace the interdependence of ALL souls as One, then peace isn't just possible, it's inevitable. This is the revolution of the soul; this is the evolution of consciousness; this is the pathway to peace.

A DIFFICULT ADMISSION

12

THIS NEXT STORY is hard for me to share. It's embarrassing because this experience happened long after I "should" have known better, long after I was already deeply immersed in service and activism and trained in recognizing the nuances of social justice. Just goes to show how difficult the process of waking up can be—it really never ends—and how quickly our deeply entrenched biases and unearned advantage can cause us to fall back asleep.

But share I must because it's a very human, quite ordinary, and utterly necessary tale to tell. It serves as an example of the thoughts and actions that have divided us, as a nation and as a people, for hundreds of years. It is also a story of self-accountability, and without that, true change can't happen. So if I really want to make a difference in the world, I must break shame and be transparent with my own fumbling humanity before I can ever encourage others to do the same.

I learned a lot in the years after I traveled to Uganda, Cambodia, and many other countries. I continued to grow and push myself to fight systems of oppression and my own complicity with them. Off the Mat evolved and began focusing more on the impact it could make at home in the United States by supporting the leadership of yogis on the margins, as well as training all yogis to use their practice to ground sustainable activism.

At this point, I was in Atlanta and had just finished teaching a large yoga event, a benefit to raise money for an organization committed to ending generational poverty among women. I had a few hours to kill before heading to the airport and was thrilled to learn my hotel wasn't far from the Martin Luther King Jr. National Historical Park, which included his childhood home; the Ebenezer Baptist Church, where he attended and preached; and Freedom Hall, where his remains are buried. I'd heard there was a man who worked at the church—an old friend of the King family—who could recite the entire "I Have a Dream" speech in Dr. King's exact rhythm and tenor. I'd been on the road for more than a month by then, teaching workshops and presenting at conferences, and I was pretty depleted. Dr. King's words would feed my soul and give me just what I needed to re-motivate and re-energize myself. I imagined sitting in a pew, in front of the pulpit where Dr. King gave his sermons, his voice beaming loud and strong to the rafters, his congregation affirming his message of love, freedom, and peace with "hallelujahs" and "amens." I was eager to pay my respects to the man who dedicated his life to civil rights and compassionate action, who inspired a movement that catalyzed social change—a movement that still exists today, albeit under different names and leadership—and whose teachings continue to inform the way justice movements organize, including the root principles of OTM.

▼

I leave the hotel and head toward the main road, which will take me to the park. It is a gorgeous day. I put my earbuds in and stroll down the avenue listening to the last speech Dr. King gave in 1968. He is talking about the story of the Good Samaritan in the Bible, about how this man was beaten by thieves and left half dead on the side of the road, and how a Levite and a priest passed right by him and did nothing to help.

"They didn't stop to help him." Dr. King's familiar and powerful voice shouts into my ears. "And finally a man of another race came by. He got down from his beast, decided not to be compassionate by proxy. But he got down with him, administered first aid, and helped the man in need. Jesus ended up saying, this was the good man, this was the great man, because he had the capacity to project the 'I' into the 'thou,' and to be concerned about his brother . . ."

I'm so completely caught up in Dr. King's speech that I don't pay much attention to my surroundings. After a bit, I look up and take stock of the neighborhood. Many stores are vacant—their windows broken and their walls overlaid with graffiti—and the apartments above them boarded up and deserted. Under worn-out canopies, dozens of homeless people take shelter from the midday sun, and a quick glance around confirms that there aren't many pedestrians besides me out and about. I'm surprised. What I imagine was once a vibrant boulevard, with bustling shops, restaurants, and residents, now seems desolate and sad. I can see Dr. King walking these very streets as a young person looking at some of the same buildings I'm looking at right now.

Dr. King's speech ends with him shouting ecstatically, "I'm not worried about anything. I'm not fearing any man! Mine eyes have seen the glory of the coming of the Lord!"

I remove my earbuds and think sadly about how prophetic a speech that was. Dr. King would be killed the very next day. I catch the eye of a woman waiting at a stop light, who is holding the hand of her young child. I smile. She nods in acknowledgment and then walks away as the light turns green. The child looks back at me curiously as they cross the street. It's only then that I realize I'm the only white person around, which suddenly makes me feel weirdly self-conscious. Like I shouldn't be here. Like I'm out of place.

By now, I've come to an underpass; it's dark and dank, and the thought of walking through it gives me pause. I look around to see if there's another way to get where I'm going, but it doesn't look like it. I take a breath and continue forward. I get about halfway through before I see a group of young men entering from the other side. Shit. I nonchalantly glance over my shoulder in hopes that someone else is behind me, but no luck. I'm definitely alone. I can feel my heart pounding and my breath getting shallow. As a woman, I'm obviously conditioned to feel concern for the safety of my body. My own history has proven that I need to be hypervigilant and cautious around men, especially when I'm walking alone. But, this time, what I feel goes beyond caution and concern. A burst of anxiety rises up as adrenaline courses through my body, signaling "danger ahead."

The men are all African American, and I am scared.

The young men, all probably in their late teens, early twenties, are talking and laughing; their voices get louder as we get closer. I purposely don't acknowledge them; I keep my head up but my gaze down toward the ground, not wanting to make eye contact. Then, with my hands by my sides, I use my thumb to turn my engagement ring around so the diamond faces my palm and can't be seen. It's a quick and instinctive move. I don't want to direct attention to anything valuable because I'm fairly certain I'm about to be robbed. Or worse. I hold my breath.

They pass me by without so much as a glance my way.

Only when I exit the tunnel do I fully exhale. My head drops in shame.

It occurs to me immediately that my reaction to those young men, and the overwhelming fear I felt in that tunnel, had to do with the color of their skin as much as it did their gender. As my heartbeat slows down and my breath returns to normal, I wonder if my experience would've been different had they been all white? Or if they had been wearing suits instead of low hung pants and hoodies? Or if I were in a "better" neighborhood? Would I have assumed that they were going to rob me then? Or rape me?

I continue walking toward Freedom Hall, acutely aware of the irony of my situation and the massive teaching that I've just been presented with. Here I am, on my way to pay my respects to the man who fought to his death for the rights of people of color, and I'm having to confront my own racism. I'm ashamed, yet it feels right that I should have to look at it in this moment.

At the park, I read and listen to the words of Dr. King, reflecting on how much has changed since he walked these streets and how much has stubbornly stayed the same. How our society is still purposely designed to establish and maintain power dynamics that elevate some and seek to tear down, alienate, and suppress others who have the same moral and constitutional rights to the society of which they are an equal part. I think about my own privilege and the ways in which I benefit from it, for no other reason than the color of my skin and my socioeconomic status. And I cringe at the thought that I considered these young men as less-thans and people to be feared. Even though I knew better. Even though I have fought for equal rights. Fuck. Institutionalized racism and ancestral bias run deep.

Standing in front of Dr. King's house, a pretty craftsman-style cottage set back from the road, I picture him on this porch as a child with his father, also a preacher, sitting nearby gently guiding him toward his future and shaping his beliefs through the word of God. The famous saying by the Australian aboriginal artist and activist Lilla Watson comes to me, and it gives me pause. "If you have come here to help me, you are wasting your time. But if you have come because your liberation is bound with mine, then let us work together." *I obviously have so much to learn*, I think to myself as I step inside the church.

At the historic Ebenezer Baptist Church, where King was baptized and eulogized, I stand solemnly in the main room where he preached, where his father and grandfather preached, and where his mother, Alberta, was assassinated. So much joy, hope, suffering, and forgiveness live in these walls. The man I had heard about, the friend of the King family, gathers a group of us around to recite "I Have a Dream." He closes his eyes, takes a breath, and begins to speak. Shivers run up and down my spine; goosebumps appear on my arms and neck. This man has captured the passion and emotion of Dr. King so well that, when I close my own eyes, I can see Dr. King standing in front of me. I try to imagine what it would've been like to have heard these words recited back in 1963. How the crowd must have stood awestruck and inspired, with absolute hope that the day would soon come when all beings, regardless of race or belief, could join together and "sing in the words of the old Negro spiritual, 'Free at last! Free at last! Thank God Almighty, we are free at last!'"

More than fifty years later, and we're still waiting.

It's time for me to get to the airport, so I leave the church and follow the same road back to the hotel that I took before. As I start back through the tunnel, I wonder how I'll react if anything comes up this time. I'm committed to being present to whatever arises. I know I must bear witness to, and transform, the deep separation that is within me if I want there to be unity for all.

As I approach the underpass, I can see another group of black men, this time standing on the corner just beyond the tunnel. I wonder what they're doing there and am dismayed that my first thought is: *They're obviously selling drugs.* I sigh. *Jesus Christ, Seane, shut up.* Just as I begin to berate myself, I hear Mona's voice, *Better out than in!* I've got to fully own my shit, without shame, otherwise I become it. I notice my body tensing up, just like before, my pulse quickening, my breath getting shorter. My anxiety increases; it's hard to stay present and focused and not let my imagination get the better of me. *Stay in your body. Feel your feet on the ground. Breathe.* I discreetly shake my hands to discharge the tension. I take a deep breath again. And then another. I keep walking.

About ten yards beyond them, I notice four men standing near a doorway; they're young cargo-pants-wearing, polo-shirted white guys. I wonder what *they're* doing in a place like this. *They must be tourists.* I don't know anything about them, but it doesn't matter. I instantly feel relief. And then shame. My heart has stopped pounding, and my breathing is slowing down; I'm much less anxious. So interesting, I think, that I feel so much safer now that I've seen those young men. My body's telling me if I can just get to where they are, I'll be out of harm's way. Why? Because they're white, and so am I? Because we're from the same "tribe"? Fuck. Now guilt adds to my shame, but I don't stop it; I let the feelings come without self-censoring.

As I reach the corner where the young black men are, one of them moves aside so that I can pass freely. A few moments later, I get to the spot where the white guys are standing, and I'm aware that I just breathed a huge sigh of relief. A short lived one, it turns out, because they immediately start harassing me. I am completely caught off guard. *Wait a minute. They're not supposed to be a threat to me—they're my people!* My body is unprepared for their verbal assault. They ask me where I'm going, what I'm doing, look me up and down suggestively, and make lewd comments. I look down at the ground, unable to respond, and feel myself dissociating, my go-to response when I'm overwhelmed. I politely ask them to let me pass. They refuse.

Just then, one of the young black men I saw on the corner approaches, interrupting the men surrounding me, and asks if I'm okay. I shake my head no.

The white foursome isn't so thrilled with the interruption and quickly walk away. The man asks where I'm headed and if he could walk with me in case those guys were still around. He's not surprised, he says, that they were giving me shit; they're from the university nearby, and they come to this neighborhood often to buy drugs.

As we walk back through the neighborhood, he tells me he's been studying at that university and plans to become a public defender so he can help those in his community— particularly African American men—get decent representation. He says it makes him angry when he sees people getting bothered like I was and that it's near impossible for him not to interfere. His mom always tells him to mind his own business, but he tells me there's no way he could live with himself if he just walked away and ignored anyone in distress.

I think of Dr. King's speech about the Good Samaritan that I listened to earlier that day "This was the good man," I heard him say, "this was the great man, because he had the capacity to project the 'I' into the 'thou,' and to be concerned about his brother." I smile.

I'm so tempted to tell him what happened to me earlier that day. How I saw these other guys coming toward me on my way to Freedom Hall and all the racist and stereotypical thoughts I had and all the assumptions I made about them and then the self-reflection that came up afterward. But I don't. It's not his job to hear my "confession" or to validate my experience or assuage my feelings of shame and guilt. Anyway, I am sure he already knows. At the hotel I shake his hand, thank him, and wish him the best at school. He smiles, tells me to stay safe, then walks away. I turn into the hotel filled with humility and gratitude. Another angel on my path. I send the young man love and wish him countless angels of his own to guide him as he makes his way through his life. May his journey be blessed.

After my experience that day in Atlanta, I called my friend Dr. Melody Moore, a faculty member of Off the Mat and a psychologist, to tell her what happened and to process what I saw as my implicit racism. I tracked in my body where the shame, fear, and deeply repressed biases and bigotry lived, breathed into it, and gave myself space to express and discharge the energy by talking it out and exploring its roots. It felt ancient and never-ending.

Melody listened patiently as I ranted. "How long have these biases lived within me? Did I inherit them? Will I ever get rid of them? And what about those young men? Had I acted on my fear, I could have put them at serious risk of harassment, jail, or even death! And what if that man didn't come to my 'rescue'? Would my opinion of him be any different? Does he suddenly become 'good' because of what he did for me? No wonder his mother tells him to mind his business. Not doing so could put her son in danger. She lives with that every day! Fuck. There is so much ignorance in the world. That's the problem, right? As long as we meet fear with fear and hate with hate, all we're doing is creating more fear, more hate, and more separation. And I just watched myself contribute to it again!"

Together we unpacked what had happened and came to the conclusion that falling into racist, classist, or any other kind of prejudiced behavior, or worrying about where it came from, isn't helpful. It is sadly a given and will continue to be as long as systems are in place to fan the flames of fear and ignorance. The bigger issue is the resistance that those of us with privilege have to looking at how our behavior and belief systems perpetuate oppression—either consciously or subconsciously—and our failure to hold ourselves accountable. So much of our biases, bigotry, and prejudice is historical, ancestral, and cultural; it informs and impacts how we live and how we relate to one another. We are taught to fear differences, instead of celebrating them; to distrust those who think, look, and act differently, rather than learning from them. All of these beliefs live in the body and, no matter how conscious we think we are, can erupt in moments of overwhelm or stress. When that happens, our own biases, ignorance, and fears rub up against someone else's. If we aren't aware of what's happening, all that rubbing creates friction, which leads to more conflict and misunderstandings, which in turn lead to pain, suffering, and even death.

In India, Uganda, Cambodia, and many other places I've visited over the years, I saw first-hand the systemic oppression born of unequal power dynamics and perpetrated through violent means that target marginalized people. The lessons I learned, the suffering I witnessed, forced me to confront the ways in which my own biases and privilege contributed to separation and oppression. Looking at all that was painful, but necessary. I knew that without doing this hard inner work, I could not be an effective and conscious changemaker.

But that day in Atlanta was different. The oppressor wasn't someone "over there" or a complex situation that I had little context for. I didn't have to travel far and wide to discover barriers to freedom. They existed, not only right in my own backyard, but right in me. I was the oppressor. I had to acknowledge the shame I felt in discovering—yet again—how deeply discrimination had taken hold in my cells. It's everywhere I look. It's everywhere I am. It's everywhere we are. Once I stepped into the tunnel, my internalized prejudice commandeered my rational mind. All the overt and the hidden bigotry I experienced within the cultural milieu of my youth—the sense of "us versus them" implied in schools, churches, and neighborhoods by white dominant culture; the stereotyping of men of color as being inherently violent and criminal; the fears and prejudices of my ancestors, which had taken root in my cells—came flooding back and landed on the shoulders of these young black men.

My experience in Atlanta was about racism. Sadly, I could have written plenty of stories about my complicity in other "isms" or phobias, too, including sexism, homophobia, transphobia, xenophobia, ableism, classism, and ageism. All of these "isms" create much division, inequality, suffering, and trauma throughout the world—and all of them are perpetuated by powerful cultural elements such as government, law, education, and media.

It's not within the scope of this book to write about the complexities of all these systems of oppression. But what I can do is reflect on my own identity as a white, privileged Western woman, and how it gives me power and makes me complicit, for example, in the systems of racism and classism. What I do know is in order to end oppression and move toward reconciliation and change, we must take accountability for our actions. In other words, for change to happen, we gotta own our own shit. And that's not easy.

But here's the thing: It really doesn't serve us to remain in denial, sitting on the prejudices we may harbor toward others because we are too ashamed or scared to admit them. They live within all of us, in different ways, imprinted deep in our cells, affecting the ways in which we see and experience the world. None of us is exempt from the insidious ways our biases keep us separate from one another and make us pawns of the systems of oppression that surround us. Consciously or unconsciously, our prejudices that support and validate this separation make us complicit in these larger systems. The good news,

however, is that each and every one of us has the power to heal the suffering we've caused and actively resist oppressive systems.

How do we do that? By taking accountability and by remembering to love. Tibyangye said it this way in Uganda: "Accountability is the key to sustainability, and compassion is the doorway to peace." Without accountability, it's too easy to blame others for the suffering we see in the world, too easy to sit back and wonder why the world is so fractured. Without compassion, we will continue to divide and fail to see the soul in all beings and the beauty in our differences. In a way, Tibyangye was telling me to come back to the essence of yoga.

Yoga as spiritual practice demands that we hold ourselves accountable for every way in which we are in service to the whole and every way in which we contribute to a fractured world. Yoga insists that we commit to the inquiry, no matter how raw, messy, or humbling it gets. And make no mistake, it takes courage and willpower because the path that leads to transformation is a long, steep, and craggy one, one that never stops unearthing the illusion of the ego and truth of the soul. It's tempting to reject such truth and surrender to the righteousness of the ego. But what then? Actually, we know exactly "what then": more division and pain. This is the state of consciousness that we are living with today as a society. And clearly, it's not working.

Looking at these uncomfortable and internalized beliefs within yourself is not a punishment; it is a gift. It means you get to grow and move toward understanding, compassion, and empathy. You get to wake up and be part of the necessary change that can ease this planet into peace. This is what you *get* to do. So you must take advantage of the spiritual tools and healing resources for transformation you have and use them. Especially if you can take action without fear of imprisonment or death—because so many people around the world cannot. Get raw, go deep, name your shadow, move beyond your limiting beliefs, confront your biases, take responsibility for the ways you're complicit in perpetrating systems of oppression, open yourself to the true power of love, speak up and out, and take action, when you can! That is yoga. That is the practice. You must do the work—we all

must—if justice and equality are ever to be possible. Remember, none of us will ever be free until all souls are free.

At first it felt like all the inner work I had done on my cushion and my mat and all the racquet smashing and emotional rinsing Mona led me through betrayed me that day in Atlanta. That it didn't prevent me from being racist. But actually, I was grateful for all those tools. As my father, who found yoga later in life, used to tell me, "It's a practice, not a perfect." The fruits of those practices brought everything to light, as it was happening, helping me see how my behavior perpetuated the very separation I abhor in our culture. I felt my shame; I saw how easily my thoughts could have become actions, which would have caused suffering in me (as the oppressor) and in those young black men (as the targets of my bigotry). I wasn't interested in glossing over my actions or even trying to defend them. I saw that, no matter how hard I tried to extinguish the ignorance and prejudices that live within me, those obstacles would keep coming back. But yoga says that's not the point. The point is I saw and felt the consequences of my actions and didn't shy away from examining them.

It's just like being in a hard yoga pose. You breathe, observe the thoughts, calm the mind, and get present to what is. In that moment of clarity, I vowed to pay even more attention to how I create harm—as a white woman of privilege in a country that lifts people up or oppresses them based on the color of their skin, the circumstances of their birth, and the amount of money they have. And I vowed to choose more loving and conscious actions. That too is yoga . . . off the mat.

The truth is the challenges don't suddenly disappear no matter how good your skills are, but the time it takes to wake up, see your part in it, and make different choices decreases. You may find yourself able to get to the truth quicker, take ownership faster, make amends, and then move on. This is the process, and the progression, that can shift the consciousness of this planet.

From all of the angels who have crossed my path and enriched my heart, I have learned that yoga is now. It's in every experience, all beings, the rising of the sun, the shifting tides, the birth, the death, and every funky, wild, and weird moment in between. It is in the beautiful and in the grotesque. It's in the broken and the healed. It is in all

souls emerging and all souls still asleep. Yoga is never an excuse to turn away from pain, discomfort, or suffering—it is an invitation to turn toward it with compassionate action. It is not a reason to bypass the heartbreak—either yours or the world's.

Yoga is what we can turn to when everything around us is falling apart, when we despair that the world will never know peace. It gives us the tools we need to pause, breathe, and listen to what wants to be known, and to move in accordance with what needs to be done for the freedom of all beings and the liberation of all souls. In that pause, we can prepare our heart to receive unconditional love and wisdom and to offer it up to all other beings. It is what reminds us that we serve others because we recognize that the Divine living in their hearts is the same essence that lives within us. Yoga is the body, it is the breath, it is the ever-evolving soul. It is the trauma, the self-discovery, the change. It is the loss, the awakening, the forgiveness. It is the love. Yoga is personal, a way to mend the fractures within yourself. But equally important, it is spiritual, a means to heal that which divides us all and to bring us back into union with each other. It is everywhere that affects the happiness and sustainability of all life. Therefore, yoga is also social, racial, and immigration justice. It is sexuality and gender justice. Disability justice. Environmental and economic justice. It is Indigenous sovereignty, animal rights, and, most certainly, politics. It's a practice of remembrance, an opportunity to shine a light on all the shattered places, and do whatever is possible to make us, each other, and this planet once again both holy and whole.

This is the revolution of the soul. It is a process of personal evolution, opening our heart to collective love, that catapults us directly into conscious, compassionate action for the good of all.

There is only one true revolution, and it begins within. End the internalized oppressive behavior by reframing the narratives we tell ourselves are true and heal from the ways that cultural, historical, generational, ancestral, and individual traumas have influenced our perception, and we will see an end to the pain and suffering that exist in the world. Why? Because when we heal the fractured parts of ourselves and learn to love who we are and the journey we've embarked upon for wholeness, we will see that same tender humanity in all souls. Doing the inner work creates compassion; it just does. Although doing the inner work is humbling and exposes the depths of our own humanity, it is only when we can be fully in the human experience and see it for what it is—a process of being that opens us, through experience, to love—that we can love all the evolving, imperfect, and wondrous souls as they come home to themselves.

So do your inner work and take action. Act as though lives depend on it, as though equality, justice, peace, and freedom depend on it. Because they do. Act like your own liberation depends on it. Because it does.

The true revolution to freedom begins, as Mona told me years ago, the moment we answer the soul's call for peace. You have been called. You have all that you need individually, we have all that we need collectively—and it is holy. So, let's wake up, remember who we really are to each other, and do whatever needs to be done now in order to create a just, equal, happy, abundant, blessed, safe, peace-filled, and loving world for *all* beings everywhere.

It's time.

EPILOGUE: THE LAST WORD

THANK YOU FOR TAKING this ride with me. It was an honor to share my stories and introduce you to the angels who have inspired my growth. In doing so, I hope I've given you the courage to unpack your own narratives, cultivate the tools to support the evolution of your soul, and work to heal any separation you might feel within yourself, toward others, or toward the planet.

May your journey be blessed, and may all souls rest, happily and easily, in unity and freedom, as the One we are, the light we've always been, and the child of God we will forever more be. For that which is within, is within all, and that which is within all is the only leader this revolution will ever need.

▼

And now, please meet one more angel.

My father was diagnosed with kidney cancer in 2003. It would take seven years and countless experiential treatments, until finally there were no more treatments to be done and no more time to be had. The cancer had taken over his body, and he was told to prepare to die.

The morning after we got the news, he and I went outside and made our way slowly across the lawn, my arm hooked around his to hold him up. His body was weak and wasted from the disease. We stood by the lake in the backyard, in silence, looking up at the rising sun. After a long while, my father spoke, without taking his eyes off the horizon. "Let me tell you a little something about life." He paused for a moment, took a breath, and continued, "It will fuck you in the ass . . ."

As I opened my mouth to protest, he put his arms around me, pulled me closer to his chest, and continued.

". . . but it will also give you this daughter to hold, and this sunrise, and more beauty than any one of us can ever possibly deserve. I'm not going to lie to you, baby, this next part is going to get rough. I know my death will be hard for you. I know it will break your heart. Let it. Let it crack you wide open. Please, for me, don't miss a moment of this. Not a single, awful, tragic second. Be with this loss, be with your grief fully. I know it will hurt, but here's the gift, and never forget this . . ."

Then he turned me around so that I could look into his eyes—blue-gray eyes with yellow around the pupil that matched mine exactly. We stared at each other for the longest time, absorbing each other into our memory. Tears began to pour out of me. He pulled me tighter to him and whispered into the side of my head.

". . . for you to hurt this badly only means you got to love that big, and if that's all you get in a single lifetime, you are more than blessed. That's all there is. Love. Let that love lead your life and your choices. Let it become who you are, and just be grateful. For all of it. Life is really hard, but it's also really good, and it's all yours, my baby. So grab it hard, hold it tight, learn all you can. Experience everything, and when it comes time to let go, like I need to now, just be thankful for it all."

He leaned down and kissed me, then said, "One day, if you ever write a book, tell them you got this from your dying dad: 'Love big, forgive always, do good, and don't be an asshole.' That's yoga, that's a life well-lived. It's really that simple. End of story."

ACKNOWLEDGMENTS

I AM BEYOND GRATEFUL for the many people who have helped make this book a reality. First, big thanks and love to everyone at Sounds True, especially Tami Simon for convincing me to stretch my self-expression beyond the yoga studio and onto the page. The three years that it took to write this book have been incredibly challenging—and wonderfully creative—and I blame Tami for all of it! Thank you Haven Iverson for your insight and skill; Rachael Murray for the cover design; Jennifer Brown, Stephen Lessard, Drummond West, and Aron Arnold for your years of love and support.

Thank you to Alex Kapitan (radicalcopyeditor.com), whose contribution as a sensitivity reader can never be overstated, and who provided the necessary guidance to synthesize complex concepts while simultaneously supporting the book's connection to Spirit. I'm so grateful for your enthusiasm, skill, and brilliance. Also, a huge shout-out to Teo Drake for providing his wisdom and insights from behind the scenes. I love you both so much!

Thank you to my dear friends Melody Moore and Kerri Kelly for being the first to read *Revolution of the Soul* way before it was ready and giving me loving but essential feedback. And to Nikki Myers, for, well, just about everything. Thank you especially to Jessica Smith, who runs my world, to Janell Cox, for being there in the early days, and to all my friends spread all over this planet. You know who you are. I treasure and love you all!

Thank you to Creative License (creativelicense.com), especially Kevin McKiernan, for working so hard and generously to secure the necessary licensing rights. Kevin, you were there from the beginning of my New York adventures and instrumental in my growth. It feels full circle to have you a part of this vision. You will always be family to me.

I am so honored that famed photographer Norman Seeff (normanseeff.com) shot me for the cover of this book. Thank you Norman for your artistry and years of friendship.

Thank you to all the many teachers, therapists, and healers I have met along the way. I can't imagine the direction my life could have gone without the support and guidance from every one of you. My commitment to your profound teachings will be to give back and share what I've learned.

Thank you to all the people who have studied with me over the years. You were all my inspiration in the writing of this book. With every word I wrote, I considered the impact it might have on your life, and when I got scared to share my vulnerability, I thought of all the ways you have shared yours with me. It gave me the courage to speak my truth in service to you. I pray your path continues to be blessed in all ways.

Thank you to Hala Khouri, Suzanne Sterling, and the Off the Mat staff, community, leaders, and faculty for the commitment you have made for inside-out social change. I am most proud of the work we have done together to raise awareness, challenge the status quo, and affirm what the power of yoga can create beyond the mat. I am truly grateful for your guidance, dedication to equity and justice, and, above all, friendship.

This book could not have been written had it not been for the brilliance, dedication, hard work, and friendship of my editor, Linda Sparrowe (lindasparrowe.com). Linda, I will forever be grateful to you. With so much patience, humor, and love, you walked me through an intimidating process, taught me how to write a book, helped me break through creative resistance, and encouraged me to tell the truth no matter what. I got so much more than an editor in you, I got a mentor, and, most importantly, a true friend for life. Thank you for having my back and for being the newest angel on my path. I love you so much.

To my entire family with infinite gratitude, with special acknowledgment to my mother Alice, my brothers Craig and Adam, my cousin Jamie, and my soul children Sophie, Ruby, and Clyde. I love you all.

Finally, to Al, my Bubbie, my heart. Thank you for your patience and for all your creative insight and contributions. I appreciate all the space you gave me to whine, moan, and complain as I figured out this mad writing process. Thank you for the kisses you doled out, the decaf soy lattes you made me, and your beautiful, tender love that wraps me in endless comfort and support. I will never take for granted how you maintain a safe, secure, grounded, quiet, drama-free, and love-filled home for us. Not only while I wrote this book, but always. I love you.

ABOUT THE AUTHOR

SEANE CORN is one of the world's most recognized yoga teachers. With her deeply passionate, often irreverent, and always inspiring presence, she has become a strong and empowered voice for personal transformation and social, environmental, and political change. In 2010, Seane was named the national yoga ambassador for YouthAIDS, an international organization that provides life-saving health services to children infected or affected by HIV/AIDS. She then cofounded Off the Mat, Into the World (OTM), which trains thousands of leaders in conscious activism worldwide, and its offshoot, the Global Seva Challenge, which raised over 3.5 million dollars for service programs in Cambodia, South Africa, Uganda, Haiti, India, Ecuador, and Kenya. In 2013, she was awarded the International Environmental Leadership Award from Global Green and honored with the Humanitarian Award from the Smithsonian Institute. In 2016, Seane went on to create the Learning and Listening Tours, traveling throughout Cuba and the United States working with progressive local leaders to share the history of systemic oppression, genocide, and racism with students and to explore what movement building for justice looks like today. Over the years, Seane has produced many top-selling and award-winning videos and DVDs, including the three-part series *The Yoga of Awakening*. *Revolution of the Soul* is her first book. Seane lives in Topanga, California, with her partner, Al, and their dog, Charlie.

ABOUT SOUNDS TRUE

SOUNDS TRUE is a multimedia publisher whose mission is to inspire and support personal transformation and spiritual awakening. Founded in 1985 and located in Boulder, Colorado, we work with many of the leading spiritual teachers, thinkers, healers, and visionary artists of our time. We strive with every title to preserve the essential "living wisdom" of the author or artist. It is our goal to create products that not only provide information to a reader or listener, but that also embody the quality of a wisdom transmission.

For those seeking genuine transformation, Sounds True is your trusted partner. At SoundsTrue.com you will find a wealth of free resources to support your journey, including exclusive weekly audio interviews, free downloads, interactive learning tools, and other special savings on all our titles.

To learn more, please visit SoundsTrue.com/freegifts or call us toll-free at 800.333.9185.

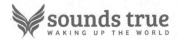